MACROECONOMICS AND HEALTH:

INVESTING IN

ECONOMIC DEVELOPMENT

"...let me say that I hope we keep our voice clear and strong on the central task of raising the health of the poor. I can be 'realistic' and 'cynical' with the best of them—giving all the reasons why things are too hard to change. We must dream a bit, not beyond the feasible but to the limits of the feasible, so that we inspire. I think that we are an important voice speaking on behalf of the world's most voiceless people today—the sick and dying among the poorest of the poor. The stakes are high. Let's therefore speak boldly so that we can feel confident that we have fulfilled our task as well as possible."

Taken by the editor from emailed correspondence from Jeffrey Sachs to the Commissioners and others working on this effort.

Information concerning the content of the report should be referred to:

Professor Jeffrey D. Sachs
Center for International Development at Harvard University
John F. Kennedy School of Government
79 John F. Kennedy Street
Cambridge, MA 02138 USA
http://www.cid.harvard.edu
jeffrey_sachs@harvard.edu

Copies of this publication can be obtained from:
World Health Organization
Marketing and Dissemination
1211 Geneva 27, Switzerland
tel: (41-22) 791 2476
fax: (41-22) 791 4857
email: bookorders@who.int

MACROECONOMICS AND HEALTH:

INVESTING IN HEALTH FOR

ECONOMIC DEVELOPMENT

REPORT OF THE COMMISSION ON MACROECONOMICS AND HEALTH

Chaired by JEFFREY D. SACHS

Presented to GRO HARLEM BRUNDTLAND,
DIRECTOR-GENERAL OF THE
WORLD HEALTH ORGANIZATION,
on 20 DECEMBER 2001

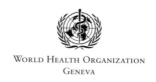

WORLD HEALTH ORGANIZATION
GENEVA

WHO Library Cataloguing-in-Publication Data

Macroeconomics and health: Investing in health for economic development.
  Report of the Commission on Macroeconomics and Health

  1.Financing, Health 2 Investments 3. Economic development
  4.Delivery of health care 5.Poverty 6.Developing countries
  7. Developed countries I.WHO Commission on Macroeconomic and Health

  ISBN 92 4 154550 X (NLM classification: WA 30)

  Second Printing

Printed in Canada
2001/13984

Editorial management: Dyna Arhin-Tenkorang, M.D., Ph.D.
Editor: Hope Steele
Design and production: Digital Design Group, Newton, MA USA

Contents

Macroeconomics and Health: Investing in Health for Economic Development

The Commission on Macroeconomics and Health (CMH) was established by World Health Organization Director-General Gro Harlem Brundtland in January 2000 to assess the place of health in global economic development. Although health is widely understood to be both a central goal and an important outcome of development, the importance of investing in health to promote economic development and poverty reduction has been much less appreciated. We have found that extending the coverage of crucial health services, including a relatively small number of specific interventions, to the world's poor could save millions of lives each year, reduce poverty, spur economic development, and promote global security.

This report offers a new strategy for investing in health for economic development, especially in the world's poorest countries, based upon a new global partnership of the developing and developed countries. Timely and bold action could save at least 8 million lives *each year* by the end of this decade, extending the life spans, productivity and economic well-being of the poor. Such an effort would require two important initiatives: a significant scaling up of the resources currently spent in the health sector by poor countries and donors alike; and tackling the non-financial obstacles that have limited the capacity of poor countries to deliver health services. We believe that the additional investments in health—requiring of donors roughly one-tenth of one percent of their national income— would be repaid many times over in millions of lives saved each year, enhanced economic development, and strengthened global security. Indeed, without such a concerted effort, the world's commitments to improving the lives of the poor embodied in the Millennium Development Goals (MDGs) cannot be met.

In many respects, the magnitude of the scaled-up effort reflects the extremely low levels of income in the countries concerned, the resulting paltry current levels of spending on health in those countries, and the costs required for even a minimally adequate level of spending on health.

Because such an ambitious effort cannot be undertaken in the health sector alone, this Report underscores the importance of an expanded aid effort to the world's poorest countries more generally. This appears to us of the greatest importance at this time, when there has been an enhanced awareness of the need to address the strains and inequities of globalization.

We call upon the world community to take heed of the opportunities for action during the coming year, by beginning the process of dramatically scaling up the access of the world's poor to essential health services. With bold decisions in 2002, the world could initiate a partnership of rich and poor of unrivaled significance, offering the gift of life itself to millions of the world's dispossessed and proving to all doubters that globalization can indeed work to the benefit of all humankind.

November 2001
Jeffrey D. Sachs, Chair
    Isher Judge Ahluwalia
    K. Y. Amoako
    Eduardo Aninat
    Daniel Cohen
    Zephirin Diabre
    Eduardo Doryan
    Richard G. A. Feachem
    Robert Fogel
    Dean Jamison
    Takatoshi Kato
    Nora Lustig
    Anne Mills
    Thorvald Moe
    Manmohan Singh
    Supachai Panitchpakdi
    Laura Tyson
    Harold Varmus

Acknowledgments

The Commissioners wish to thank WHO Director-General Dr. Gro Harlem Brundtland for her vision in establishing and actively supporting the work of the Commission. Vital support came from all of the Working Group Chairs, and the Commissioners wish to acknowledge the extraordinary work of Chairs Isher Judge Alhuwalia, George Alleyne, Kwesi Botchwey, Daniel Cohen, Zephirin Diabre, Richard Feachem, Prabhat Jha, Chris Lovelace, Anne Mills, Carin Norberg, and Alan Tait. WHO executive directors and senior policy advisors to the Director-General also made invaluable inputs. The Commissioners are also indebted to the members of the Working Groups and the authors of the commissioned papers, whose names are listed in the Acknowledgments. Dyna Arhin-Tenkorang served skillfully as Senior Economist and Special Assistant to the Chairman. Technical assistance and help in the drafting of the Report also came from hundreds of dedicated individuals around the world. Among the many individuals who devoted especially long hours to the preparation of the Report, we would like to pay special thanks to Peter Heller, Paul Isenman, Inge Kaul, and Susan Stout.

The WHO Secretariat, led by Sergio Spinaci, with able assistance provided by Eveline Coveney, Aquilina John-Mutaboyerwa, and Elisa Pepe, skillfully supported the Project in every way. The Commissioners also gratefully acknowledge the editorial assistance in the preparation of the Report of Hope Steele and Marc Kaufman.

The Commission gratefully acknowledges the financial support provided by the Bill and Melinda Gates Foundation, the United Kingdom Department for International Development, the Grand Duchy of Luxembourg, the Government of Ireland, the Government of Norway, the Rockefeller Foundation, the Government of Sweden, and the United Nations Foundation.

EXECUTIVE SUMMARY OF THE REPORT

Technology and politics have thrust the world more closely together than ever before. The benefits of globalization are potentially enormous, as a result of the increased sharing of ideas, cultures, life-saving technologies, and efficient production processes. Yet globalization is under trial, partly because these benefits are not yet reaching hundreds of millions of the world's poor, and partly because globalization introduces new kinds of international challenges as turmoil in one part of the world can spread rapidly to others, through terrorism, armed conflict, environmental degradation, or disease, as demonstrated by the dramatic spread of AIDS around the globe in a single generation.

The world's political leaders have recognized this global interdependence in solemn commitments to improve the lives of the world's poor by the year 2015. The Millennium Development Goals (MDGs), adopted at the Millennium Summit of the United Nations in September 2000, call for a dramatic reduction in poverty and marked improvements in the health of the poor. Meeting these goals is feasible but far from automatic. Indeed, on our current trajectory, those goals will not be met for a significant proportion of the world's poor. Success in achieving the MDGs will require a seriousness of purpose, a political resolve, and an adequate flow of resources from high-income to low-income countries on a sustained and well-targeted basis.

The importance of the MDGs in health is, in one sense, self-evident. Improving the health and longevity of the poor is an end in itself, a fundamental goal of economic development. But it is also a *means* to achieving the other development goals relating to poverty reduction. The linkages of health to poverty reduction and to long-term economic growth are powerful, much stronger than is generally understood. The burden of disease in some low-income regions, especially sub-Saharan Africa, stands as a stark barrier to economic growth and therefore must be addressed frontally and centrally in any comprehensive development strategy. The AIDS pandemic represents a unique challenge of unprecedented urgency and intensity. This single epidemic can undermine Africa's development over the next generation, and may cause tens of millions of deaths in

Table 1. LIFE EXPECTANCY AND MORTALITY RATES, BY COUNTRY DEVELOPMENT CATEGORY, (1995–2000)

Development Category	Population (1999 millions)	Annual Average Income (US dollars)	Life Expectancy at Birth (years)	Infant Mortality (deaths before age 1 per 1,000 live births)	Under Five Mortality (deaths before age 5 per 1,000 live births)
Least-Developed Countries	643	296	51	100	159
Other Low-Income Countries	1,777	538	59	80	120
Lower-Middle-Income Countries	2,094	1,200	70	35	39
Upper-Middle-Income Countries	573	4,900	71	26	35
High-Income Countries	891	25,730	78	6	6
Memo: sub-Saharan Africa	642	500	51	92	151

Source: Human Development Report 2001, Table 8, and CMH calculations using World Development Indicators of the World Bank, 2001.

India, China, and other developing countries unless addressed by greatly increased efforts.

Our Report focuses mainly on the low-income countries and on the poor in middle-income countries.[1] The low-income countries, with 2.5 billion people—and especially the countries in sub-Saharan Africa, with 650 million people—have far lower life expectancies and far higher age-adjusted mortality rates than the rest of the world, as shown in the accompanying Table 1. The same is true for the poor in middle-income countries, such as China. To reduce these staggeringly high mortality rates, the control of communicable diseases and improved maternal and child health remain the highest public health priorities. The main causes of avoidable deaths in the low-income countries are HIV/AIDS, malaria, tuberculosis (TB), childhood infectious diseases, maternal and perinatal conditions, micronutrient deficiencies, and tobacco-related illnesses. If these conditions were controlled in conjunction with enhanced programs of family planning, impoverished families could not only enjoy lives that are longer, healthier, and more productive, but they would also choose to have fewer children, secure in the knowledge that their children would survive, and could thereby invest more in the education and health of each child. Given the special burdens of some of these conditions on women, the well-being of women would especially be improved. The improvements in health would translate into higher incomes, higher economic growth, and reduced population growth.

Even though we focus mainly on communicable diseases and maternal and perinatal health, noncommunicable diseases (NCDs) are also of great significance for all developing countries; for many middle-income countries the mortality from communicable diseases has already been significantly reduced so that the NCDs tend to be the highest priority. Many of the noncommunicable diseases, including cardiovascular disease, diabetes, mental illnesses, and cancers, can be effectively addressed by relatively low-cost interventions, especially using preventative actions relating to diet, smoking, and lifestyle.[2] Our global perspective on priorities needs to be complemented by each country analyzing its own health priorities based on detailed and continually updated epidemiological evidence. Our argument for outcome-oriented health systems also implies substantial capacity to deal with a range of conditions not detailed here, such as low-cost case-management of mental illness, diabetes and heart attacks. The evidence also suggests that approaches required to scale up the health system to provide interventions for communicable diseases and reproductive health will also improve care for the NCDs.[3]

The feasibility of meeting the MDGs in the low-income countries is widely misjudged. On the one side of the debate are those optimists who believe that the health goals will take care of themselves, as a fairly automatic byproduct of economic growth. With the mortality rates of children under 5 in the least-developed countries standing at 159 per 1,000 births, compared with 6 per 1,000 births in the high-income countries,[4] these blithe optimists assume that it's just a matter of time before the mortality rates in the low-income world will converge with those of the rich countries. This is false for two reasons. First, the disease burden itself will slow the economic growth that is presumed to solve the health problems; second, economic growth is indeed important, but is very far from enough. Health indicators vary widely for the same income level. The evidence suggests that 73 countries are far behind in meeting the MDGs for infant mortality, and 66 are far behind for meeting the MDGs for child mortality.[5] The disease burden can be brought down in line with the MDGs only if there is a concerted, global strategy of increasing the access of the world's poor to essential health services.

On the other side of the debate are the pessimists, who underestimate the considerable progress that has been made in health (with the notable exception of HIV/AIDS) by most low-income countries and believe that their remaining high disease burden is a byproduct of corrupt and broken health systems beyond repair in poorly governed low-income countries. This alternative view is also filled with misunderstanding and exaggeration. The epidemiological evidence conveys a crucial message: the vast majority of the excess disease burden is the result of a relatively small number of identifiable conditions, each with a set of existing health interventions that can dramatically improve health and reduce the deaths associated with these conditions. The problem is that these interventions don't reach the world's poor. Some of the reasons for this are corruption, mismanagement, and a weak public sector, but in the vast majority of countries, there is a more basic and remediable problem. The poor lack the financial resources to obtain coverage of these essential interventions, as do their governments. In many cases, public health programs have not been modified to focus on the conditions and interventions emphasized here.

The key recommendation of the Commission is that the world's low- and middle-income countries, in partnership with high-income countries, should scale up the access of the world's poor to essential health services, including a focus on specific interventions. The low- and middle-income countries would commit additional domestic financial resources, political leadership, transparency, and systems for community involvement and accountability, to ensure that adequately financed health systems can operate effectively and are dedicated to the key health problems. The high-income countries would simultaneously commit vastly increased financial assistance, in the form of grants, especially to the countries that need help most urgently, which are concentrated in sub-Saharan Africa. *They would resolve that lack of donor funds should not be the factor that limits the capacity to provide health services to the world's poorest peoples.*

The partnership would need to proceed step by step, with actions in the low-income countries creating the conditions for donor financing, while ample donor financing creates the financial reality for a greatly scaled-up, more effective health system, with the shared program subject to frequent review, evaluation, verification, and mid-course corrections. The chicken-and-egg problem of deciding whether reform or donor financing must come first would be put aside with both donors and recipients frankly acknowledging that both finance and reform are needed at each stage, and that both must be sustained by an intensive partnership. For lower-middle-income countries with large concentrations of poor, a prime task of national governments would be to mobilize additional resources to finance priority interventions that assure coverage of the poor within those societies.

The commitment of massive additional financial resources for health, domestic and international, may be a necessary condition for scaling up health interventions, but the Commission recognizes that such a commitment will not be sufficient. Past experience shows compellingly that political and administrative commitments on the part of both donors and countries are key to success. Building health systems that are responsive to client needs, particularly for poor and hard-to-reach populations, requires politically difficult and administratively demanding choices. Some issues, such as relative commitments to the health needs of rich and poor, relate to the health sector. Others, such as whether the public sector budget and procurement systems work or whether there is effective supervision and local accountability of public service delivery, are public management issues. Underlying these issues are broader questions of governance, conflict, and the relative importance of development and poverty reduction in national priorities.

The Commission recognizes the importance of these and other constraints and treats them in depth in several places in this Report. Success will require strong political leadership and commitment on the part of countries that can afford to contribute resources as well as from developing countries—in the private and public sectors and in civil society as well. It requires the evolution of an atmosphere of honesty, trust, and respect in donor-recipient interactions. Success requires special efforts precisely in those settings in which health conditions are most troubling and where public sectors are weak. Donor support should be readily forthcoming to help overcome these constraints. Where countries are not willing to make a serious effort, though, or where funding is misused, prudence and credibility require that large-scale funding should not be provided. Even here, though, the record shows that donor assistance can do much to help, by building local capacity and through the involvement of civil society and NGOs. This is a daunting challenge, yet one that is more than ever a strategically relevant objective. Governments and leaders who help stimulate and nurture these actions will be providing a specific antidote to the despair and hatred that poverty can breed.

The Commission worked hard to examine whether the low-income countries could afford to fund the health systems out of their own resources if they were to eliminate existing wasteful spending in health and other areas. Our findings are clear: *poverty itself imposes a basic financial constraint, though waste does exist and needs to be addressed.* The poor countries should certainly improve health-sector management, review the current balance among health-sector programs, and raise domestic resources for health within their limited means. We believe that it is feasible, on average, for low- and middle-income countries to increase budgetary outlays for health by 1 percent of GNP by 2007 and 2 percent of GNP by 2015 compared with current levels, though this may be optimistic given intense competing demands for scarce public resources. Low- and middle-income countries could also do more to make the current spending, public and private, more equitable and effective. Public spending should be better targeted to the poor, with priorities set on the basis of epidemiological and economic evidence. There is scope for private out-of-pocket spending in some cases being replaced with prepaid community financing schemes. Yet for the low-income countries, we still find a gap between financial means and financial needs, which can be filled only by the donor world if there is to be any hope of success in meeting the MDGs.

In most middle-income countries, average health spending per person is already adequate to ensure universal coverage for essential interventions. Yet such coverage does not reach many of the poor. Exclusion is often concentrated by region (e.g., rural western China and rural northeast Brazil), or among ethnic and racial minorities. For whatever reason, public-sector spending on health does not attend sufficiently to the needs of the poor. Moreover, since many middle-income countries provide inadequate financial protection for large portions of their population, catastrophic medical expenses impoverish many households. In view of the adverse consequences of ill health on overall economic development and poverty reduction, we strongly urge the middle-income countries to undertake fiscal and organizational reforms to ensure universal coverage for priority health interventions.[6] We also believe that the World Bank and the regional development banks, through nonconcessional financing, can help these countries to make a multi-year transition to universal coverage for essential health services.

The Commission examined the evidence relating to organizational requirements for scaling up and some of the key constraints that will have to be overcome. Fortunately, the essential interventions highlighted here are generally not technically exacting. Few require hospitals. Most can be delivered at health centers, at smaller facilities that we refer to as health posts, or through outreach services from these facilities. We call these collectively the *close-to-client (CTC)* system, and this system should be given priority to make these interventions widely accessible. Producing an effective CTC system is no small task. National leadership, coupled with capacity and accountability at the local level, is vital. This will require new political commitments, increased organizational and supervisory capacity at both local and higher levels, and greater transparency in public services and budgeting—all backed by more funding. These, in turn, must be built on a foundation of strong community-level oversight and action, in order to be responsive to the poor, in order to build accountability of local services, and in order to help ensure that families take full advantage of the services provided.

Some recent global initiatives for disease control, including those for TB, leprosy, guinea-worm disease, and Chagas disease, have proved highly successful in delivering quality interventions and, in some cases, changing attitudes and behaviors in some very difficult situations over large geographical areas. An important feature of these initiatives is the inclusion of rigorous systems of monitoring, evaluation, reporting, and financial control as mechanisms for ensuring that objectives are met, problems are detected and corrected, and resources are fully accountable. The result is a growing body of evidence concerning both the degree of progress achieved and the operational and managerial strategies that contribute to success. Lessons from these experiences can provide useful operational guidance, especially for the delivery of interventions at the close-to-client level.

In most countries, the CTC system would involve a mix of state and nonstate health service providers, with financing guaranteed by the state. The government may directly own and operate service units, or may contract for services with for-profit and not-for-profit providers. Since public health systems in poor countries have been so weak and underfinanced in recent years, a considerable nongovernmental health sector has arisen that is built upon private practice, religiously affiliated providers, and nongovernmental organizations. This variety of providers is useful in order to provide competition and a safety valve in case of failure of the public system. It is also a fait accompli in almost all poor countries.

A sound global strategy for health will also invest in new knowledge. One critical area of knowledge investment is operational research regarding treatment protocols in low-income countries.[7] There is still much to be learned about what actually works, and why or why not, in many low-income settings, especially where interventions have not been used or documented to date. Even when the basic technologies of disease control are clear and universally applicable, each local setting poses special problems of logistics, adherence, dosage, delivery, and drug formulation that must be uncovered through operational research at the local level. We recommend that as a normal matter, country-specific projects should allocate at least 5 percent of all resources to project-related operational research in order to examine efficacy, the optimization of treatment protocols, the economics of alternative interventions, and delivery modes and population/patient preferences.

There is also an urgent need for investments in new and improved technologies to fight the killer diseases. Recent advances in genomics, for example, bring us much closer to the long-sought vaccines for malaria and HIV/AIDS, and lifetime protection against TB. The science remains complex, however, and the outcomes unsure. The evidence suggests high social returns to investments in research that are far beyond current levels. Whether or not effective vaccines are produced, new drugs will certainly be needed, given the relentless increase of drug-resistant strains of disease agents. The Commission therefore calls for a significant scaling up of financing for global R&D on the heavy disease burdens of the poor. We draw particular attention to the diseases overwhelmingly concentrated in poor countries. For these diseases, the rich-country markets offer little incentive for R&D to cover the relatively few cases that occur in these rich countries.[8] We also stress the need for research into reproductive health—for example, new microbicides that could block the transmission of HIV/AIDS and improved management of life-threatening obstetric conditions.

We need increased investments in other areas of knowledge as well. Basic and applied scientific research in the biomedical and health sciences in the low-income countries needs to be augmented, in conjunction with increased R&D aimed at specific diseases. The state of epidemiological knowledge—who suffers and dies and of which diseases—must be greatly enhanced, through improved surveillance and reporting systems.[9] In public health, such knowledge is among the most important tools available to successful disease control. Surveillance is also critically needed in the case of many NCDs, including mental health, the impact of violence and accidents, and the rapid rise of tobacco and diet/nutrition-related diseases.

Finally, we need a greatly enhanced system of advising and training throughout the low-income countries, so that the lessons of experience in one country can be mobilized elsewhere. The international diffusion of new knowledge and "best practices" is one of the key forces of scaling up, a central responsibility of organizations such as the World Health Organization and the World Bank, and a goal now more readily achieved through low-cost methods available through the internet.

A war against disease requires not only financial resources, sufficient technology, and political commitment, but also a strategy, operational lines of responsibility, and the capacity to learn along the way. The Commission therefore devoted substantial effort to analyzing the organizational practicalities of a massive, donor-supported scaling up of health interventions in the low-income world. We started by noting the changes that will be needed on the ground within the countries themselves. After all, essential health interventions are delivered in the communities where poor people live. Scaling up must therefore start with the organization of the CTC delivery system at the local level. The role of community involvement, and more generally of mobilization of a broad partnership of public and private sectors and civil society, is crucial here. The CTC system should also be supported by nationwide programs for some major diseases, such as malaria, HIV/AIDS, and TB. Such focused programs have important advantages when properly integrated with community health delivery, by mobilizing communities of expertise not available at the community level, public attention and financing, political energies, and public accountability for specified results.

Since scaling up will require a significant increase in international financing, an effective partnership of donors and recipient countries, based on mutual trust and performance, is essential. In this context, the mechanisms of donor financing must change, a point that has been recognized in the international system in the past 3 years by the creative introduction of a new framework for poverty reduction, often termed the *Poverty Reduction Strategy Paper (PRSP) framework*.[10] The early results of the PRSP process to date are promising, and the Commission endorses this new process.[11] A concerted attack on disease along the lines that we recommend will help to ensure success of this emerging approach to donor–recipient relations. The strengths of the PRSP include: (1) deeper debt cancellation, (2) country leadership in the preparation of the national strategy, (3) explicit incorporation of civil society at each step of the process, (4) a comprehensive approach to poverty reduction, and (5) more donor coordination in support of country goals. All of these are applicable—indeed vital—to the success of the health initiative proposed here. To achieve the potential benefits of the PRSP framework, donor and recipient countries must specify a sustainable financing scheme and investment plan for the health sector as an integral part of the PRSP scheme for health.

Though we advocate a greatly increased investment in the health sector itself, we stress the need for complementary additional investments in areas with an important impact on poverty alleviation (including effects on health). These include education, water and sanitation, and agricultural improvement. For example, education is a key determinant of health status, as health is of education status. Investments in these various sectors work best when made in combination, a point highlighted by the PRSP process. We did not, however, make cost estimates outside of the health sector.[12]

Within the context of the PRSP, the Commission recommends that each developing country establish a temporary National Commission on Macroeconomics and Health (NCMH), or its equivalent, chaired jointly by the Ministers of Health and Finance and incorporating key representatives of civil society, to organize and lead the task of scaling up.[13] Each NCMH would assess national health priorities, establish a multi-year strategy to extend coverage of essential health services, take account of synergies with other key health producing sectors, and ensure consistency with a sound macroeconomic policy framework. The plan would be predicated upon greatly expanded international grant assistance. The National Commissions would work together with the WHO and World Bank to prepare an epidemiological baseline, quantified operational targets, and a medium-term financing plan. Each Commission should complete its work within two years, by the end of 2003.

We recommend that each country will need to define an overall program of "essential interventions" to be guaranteed universal coverage through public (plus donor) financing. We suggest four main criteria in choosing these essential interventions: (1) they should be technically efficacious and can be delivered successfully; (2) the targeted diseases should impose a heavy burden on society, taking into account individual illness as well as social spillovers (such as epidemics and adverse economic effects); (3) social benefits should exceed costs of the interventions (with benefits including life-years saved and spillovers such as fewer orphans or faster economic growth); and (4) the needs of the poor should be stressed.

We estimate that by 2010 around 8 million lives *per year,* in principle, could be saved—mainly in the low-income countries—by the essential interventions against infectious diseases and nutritional deficiencies recommended here.[14] The CMH estimated the costs of this expanded coverage,[15] including related general costs of system expansion and supervision, for all countries with 1999 GNP per capita below $1,200, plus the remaining handful of countries in sub-Saharan Africa with incomes above $1,200 (see Table A2.B for the list of countries).[16] Total annual health outlays for this group of countries would rise by $57 billion by 2007 and by $94 billion by 2015 (Table A2.3). The countries in the aggregate would commit an additional $35 billion per year by 2007 and $63 billion per year by 2015.[17] The donors, on their part, would contribute grant financing of an additional $22 billion per year by 2007 and $31 billion per year by 2015 (Table A2.6).[18] Current official development assistance (ODA) is on the order of $6 billion.[19] Total donor spending, including both country-level programs and the supply of global public goods, would be $27 billion in 2007 and $38 billion in 2015. The increased donor financing for health would be additional to overall current aid flows, since aid should be increased in many areas outside of the health sector as well.

Most of the donor assistance would be directed at the least-developed countries, which need the most grant assistance to extend the coverage of health services. For those countries, total annual health outlays would rise by $17 billion by 2007 and $29 billion by 2015, above the level of 2002. Given the extremely low incomes in these countries, domestic resource mobilization would fall far short of need, however, rising by $4 billion by 2007 and $9 billion by 2015. The gap would be filled by donors, with grant assistance equal to $14 billion per year in 2007 and $21 billion per year in 2015. We also note that, on a regional basis, Africa would receive the largest proportion of donor assistance, a reflection both of Africa's poverty and its high disease prevalence. AIDS prevention and care would account for around half of the total cost of scaling up.[20]

To understand these sums, it is instructive to consider the costs of the health interventions on a per capita basis. We find that, on average, the set of essential interventions costs around $34 per person per year, a very modest sum indeed, especially compared with average per capita health spending in the high-income countries of more than $2,000 per year. The least developed countries can mobilize around $15 per person per year by 2007 (almost 5 percent of per capita income). The gap is therefore $19 per person per year. With 750 million people in the least-developed countries in 2007, that comes to around $14 billion. The other low-income countries can mobilize around $32 per person on average (again roughly 5 percent of per capita income). Some of these countries will need donor aid to reach the $34 per person requirement, and others will not. The other low-income countries will have a combined population of around 2 billion in 2007, and when calculated on a country-by-country basis will need roughly $3 per capita on average to close the financing gap, therefore requiring a total level of donor aid of approximately $6 billion. The low-middle-income countries will need an additional $1.5 billion, mainly to cover the high costs of AIDS.

It is important to put the total donor assistance into perspective. Although the required assistance is large relative to current donor assistance in health, it would be only around 0.1 percent of donor GNP, and would leave ample room for significant increases in other areas of donor assistance as needed. We stress that the increased aid for health must be additional to current aid flows, since indeed increased aid will be needed not only in health but also in education, sanitation, water supply, and other areas. Also, although the donor flows look large in relation to current health spending, particularly in the poorest countries, this reflects how little they spend, which in turn reflects their low incomes. This expansion of aid to the health sector needs to be phased over time to ensure that resources are used effectively and honestly, which led us to the time path of increasing coverage shown in Table 7, which shows the basis of our costing. Note that the donor assistance will be required for a sustained period of time, perhaps 20 years, but will eventually phase out as countries achieve higher per capita incomes and are thereby increasingly able to cover essential health services out of their own resources.

This program would yield economic benefits vastly greater than its costs. Eight million lives saved from infectious diseases and nutritional deficiencies would translate into a far larger number of *years* of life saved for those affected, as well as a higher quality of life. Economists talk of disability-adjusted life years (DALYs) saved,[21] which add together the increased years of life and the reduced years of living with disabilities. We estimate that approximately 330 million DALYs would be saved for each 8 million deaths prevented. Assuming, conservatively, that each DALY saved gives an economic benefit of 1 year's per capita income of a projected $563 in 2015, the direct economic benefit of saving 330 million DALYs would be $186 billion per year, and plausibly several times that.[22] Economic growth would also accelerate, and thereby the saved

DALYs would help to break the poverty trap that has blocked economic growth in high-mortality low-income countries. This would add tens or hundreds of billions of dollars more per year through increased per capita incomes.

The $27 billion of total grant assistance in 2007 would be devoted to three goals: (1) assistance to low-income countries (and to a few middle-income countries for HIV/AIDS-related expenditures) to help pay for the scaling up of essential interventions and health system development ($22 billion, detailed in Appendix 2); (2) investments in research and development (R&D) devoted to the diseases of the poor ($3 billion); and (3) increased delivery of global public goods by the international institutions charged with coordinating the global effort, including the World Health Organization, the World Bank, and other specialized United Nations agencies ($2 billion). There would also be additional nonconcessional loan assistance for middle-income countries.[23] We believe that if well managed and phased in along the timetable that we recommend, these requisite flows could be absorbed by the developing countries without undue macroeconomic or sectoral destabilization.

These financial targets are a vision of what should be done, rather than a prediction of what will happen. We are all too aware of donor countries that neglect their international obligations despite vast wealth, and of recipient countries that abjure the governance needed to save their own people. Maybe little increased funding will take place; donors might give millions when billions are needed, and impoverished countries will fight wars against people rather than disease, making it impossible for the world community to help. We are not naïve: it is no accident that millions of people—voiceless, powerless, unnoticed by the media—die unnecessarily every year.[24]

The delivery of such large donor financing will require a new *modus operandi*. The Commission strongly supports the establishment of the Global Fund to Fight AIDS, Tuberculosis, and Malaria (GFATM), which initially will focus on the global response to AIDS, malaria, and TB. We recommend that the GFATM be scaled up to around $8 billion per year by 2007 as part of the overall $22 billion of donor aid to country programs. Given the unique challenge posed by AIDS and its capacity to overturn economic development in Africa and other regions for decades, we believe that the GFATM should support a bold and aggressive program that focuses on prevention of new infections together with treatment for those already infected. Prevention efforts would aim at achieving a high coverage of prevention programs for highly vulnerable groups including commercial sex workers and injection drug users, and achieving widespread access to treatment of sexually transmitted infections (STIs), voluntary counseling and testing (VCT), and interventions to interrupt mother-to-child transmission. Given the costs and challenges of scaling up treatment, especially using antiretroviral therapy (ART) effectively and without promoting viral resistance to the drugs, scaling up should be carefully monitored, science-based, and subject to intensive operational research. We endorse the estimates of UNAIDS and WHO's ART program that 5 million people can be brought under antiretroviral treatment in low-income settings by the end of 2006.[25]

To help channel the increased R&D outlays, we endorse the establishment of a new Global Health Research Fund (GHRF), with disbursements of around $1.5 billion per year. This fund would support basic and applied biomedical and health sciences research on the health problems affecting the world's poor and on the health systems and policies needed to address them. Another $1.5 billion per year of R&D support should be funded through existing channels. These include the Special Programme for Research and Training in Tropical Diseases (TDR), the Initiative for Vaccine Research (IVR), the Special Programme of Research, Development and Research Training in Human Reproduction (HRP) (all housed at WHO) and the public-private partnerships for AIDS, TB, malaria, and other disease control programs that have recently been established. In both cases, the predictability of increased funding would be vital, as the necessary R&D undertakings are long-term ventures. The existing Global Forum for Health Research could play an important role in the effective allocation of this overall assistance. To support this increased research and development, we strongly advocate the free internet-based dissemination of leading scientific journals, thereby increasing the access of scientists in the low-income countries to a vital scientific research tool.

The public sector cannot bear this burden on its own. The pharmaceutical industry must be a partner in this effort. The corporate principles that have spurred recent and highly laudable programs of drug donations and price discounts need to be generalized to support the scaling up of health interventions in the poor countries. The pharmaceutical industry needs to ensure that low-income countries (and the donors on their behalf) have access to essential medicines at near-production cost (sometimes termed the *lowest viable commercial price*) rather than the much higher prices that are typical of high-income markets. Industry is ready, in our estimation, for such a commitment, enabling access of the poor to essential medicines, both through differential pricing and licensing their products to generics producers.[26] If industry cooperation is not enough or not forthcoming on a general and reliable basis, the rules of international trade involving access to essential medicines should be applied in a manner that ensures the same results. At the same time, it is vital to ensure that increased access for the poor does not undermine the stimulus to future innovation that derives from the system of intellectual property rights. Private industry outside of the pharmaceutical sector also has a role to play, including by ensuring that their own labor force—the heart of a firm's productivity—has access to the knowledge and medical services that ensure their survival and health. For example, the mining companies of southern Africa, at the epicenter of HIV/AIDS, have a special responsibility to help prevent transmission and to work with government and donors to ensure that their workers have access to care. The main findings of the Commission regarding the links of health and development are summarized in Table 2. An action agenda is summarized in Table 3. Our specific recommendations on increased international donor assistance and domestic financing are summarized in Table 4.

With globalization on trial as never before, the world must succeed in achieving its solemn commitments to reduce poverty and improve health. The resources—human, scientific, and financial—exist to succeed, but now must be mobilized. As the world embarks on a heightened struggle against the evils of terrorism, it is all the more important that the world simultaneously commit itself to sustaining millions of lives through peaceful means as well, using the best of our modern science and technology and the enormous wealth of the rich countries. This would be an effort that would inspire and unite peoples all over the world. We call upon the leaders of the international community—in donor and recipient nations, in international institutions such as the World Bank, the World Health Organization, the World Trade Organization, the Organisation for Economic Co-operation and Development, and the International Monetary Fund, in private enterprise, and in civil society—to seize the opportunities identified in this report. Now, united, the world can initiate and facilitate the global investments in health that can transform the lives and livelihoods of the world's poor.

Table 2. KEY FINDINGS ON THE LINKAGES OF HEALTH AND DEVELOPMENT

1. Health is a priority goal in its own right, as well as a central input into economic development and poverty reduction. The importance of investing in health has been greatly underestimated, not only by analysts but also by developing-country governments and the international donor community. Increased investments in health as outlined in this Report would translate into hundreds of billions of dollars per year of increased income in the low-income countries. There are large social benefits to ensuring high levels of health coverage of the poor, including spillovers to wealthier members of the society.

2. A few health conditions are responsible for a high proportion of the health deficit: HIV/AIDS, malaria, TB, childhood infectious diseases (many of which are preventable by vaccination), maternal and perinatal conditions, tobacco-related illnesses, and micronutrient deficiencies. Effective interventions exist to prevent and treat these conditions. Around 8 million deaths per year from these conditions could be averted by the end of the decade in a well-focused program.

3. The HIV/AIDS pandemic is a distinct and unparalleled catastrophe in its human dimension and its implications for economic development. It therefore requires special consideration. Tried and tested interventions within the health sector are available to address most of the causes of the health deficit, including HIV/AIDS.

4. Investments in reproductive health, including family planning and access to contraceptives, are crucial accompaniments of investments in disease control. The combination of disease control and reproductive health is likely to translate into reduced fertility, greater investments in the health and education of each child, and reduced population growth.

5. The level of health spending in the low-income countries is insufficient to address the health challenges they face. We estimate that minimum financing needs to be around $30 to $40 per person per year to cover essential interventions, including those needed to fight the AIDS pandemic, with much of that sum requiring budgetary rather than private-sector financing. Actual health spending is considerably lower. The least-developed countries average approximately $13 per person per year in total health expenditures, of which budgetary outlays are just $7. The other low-income countries average approximately $24 per capita per year, of which budgetary outlays are $13.

6. Poor countries can increase the domestic resources that they mobilize for the health sector and use those resources more efficiently. Even with more efficient allocation and greater resource mobilization, the levels of funding necessary to cover essential services are far beyond the financial means of many low-income countries, as well as a few middle-income countries with high prevalence of HIV/AIDS.

7. Donor finance will be needed to close the financing gap, in conjunction with best efforts by the recipient countries themselves. We estimate that a worldwide scaling up of health investments for the low-income countries to provide the essential interventions of $30 to 40 per person will require approximately $27 billion per year in donor grants by 2007, compared with around $6 billion per year that is currently provided. This funding should be additional to other donor financing, since increased aid is also needed in other related areas such as education, water, and sanitation.

8. Increased health coverage of the poor would require greater financial investments in specific health sector interventions, as well as a properly structured health delivery system that can reach the poor. The highest priority is to create a service delivery system at the local ("close-to-client") level, complemented by nationwide programs for some major diseases. Successful implementation of such a program requires political and administrative commitment, strengthening of country technical and administrative expertise, substantial strengthening of public management systems, and creation of systems of community accountability. It also requires new approaches to donor/recipient relations.

9. An effective assault on diseases of the poor will also require substantial investments in global public goods, including increased collection and analysis of epidemiological data, surveillance of infectious diseases, and research and development into diseases that are concentrated in poor countries (often, though not exclusively, tropical diseases).

10 Coordinated actions by the pharmaceutical industry, governments of low-income countries, donors, and international agencies are needed to ensure that the world's low-income countries have reliable access to essential medicines.

Table 3.   AN ACTION AGENDA FOR INVESTING IN HEALTH FOR
ECONOMIC DEVELOPMENT

1. Each low- and middle-income country should establish a temporary National
    Commission on Macroeconomics and Health (NCMH), or its equivalent, to formulate
    a long-term program for scaling up essential health interventions as part of their over-
    all framework in their Poverty Reduction Strategy Paper (PRSP). The WHO and the
    World Bank should assist national Commissions to establish epidemiological base-
    lines, operational targets, and a framework for long-term donor financing. The
    NCMHs should complete their work by the end of 2003.

2. The financing strategy should envisage an increase of domestic budgetary resources
    for health of 1 percent of GNP by 2007 and 2 percent of GNP by 2015 (or less, if a
    smaller increase is sufficient to cover the costs of scaling up, as may be true in some
    middle-income countries). For low-income countries, this entails an additional budget-
    ary outlay of $23 billion by 2007 and $40 billion by 2015, of which the least-devel-
    oped countries account for $4 billion by 2007 and $9 billion by 2015 themselves, and
    the other low-income countries the balance. Countries should also take steps to
    enhance the efficiency of domestic resource spending, including a better prioritization
    of health services and the encouragement of community-financing schemes to ensure
    improved risk pooling for poor households.

3. The international donor community should commit adequate grant resources for low-
    income countries to ensure universal coverage of essential interventions as well as
    scaled-up R&D and other public goods. A few middle-income countries will also
    require grant assistance to meet the financial costs of expanded HIV/AIDS control.
    According to our estimates, total needs for donor grants will be $27 billion per year
    in 2007 and $38 billion per year in 2015. In addition, the World Bank and the region-
    al development banks should offer increased nonconcessional loans to middle-income
    countries aiming to upgrade their health systems. The allocation of donor commit-
    ments would be roughly as follows:

	2007	2015
Country-level programs	$22 billion	$31 billion
R&D for diseases of the poor	$3 billion	$4 billion
Provision of other Global Public Goods	$2 billion	$3 billion
Total	$27 billion	$38 billion

The WHO and the World Bank, with a steering committee of donor and recipient
countries, should be charged with coordinating and monitoring the resource mobilization process. Implementing this vision of greatly expanded support for health requires
donor support for build-up of implementation capacity and for addressing governance
or other constraints. Where funds are not used appropriately, however, credibility
requires that funding be cut back and used to support capacity building and NGO
programs.

4. The international community should establish two new funding mechanisms, with the following approximate scale of annual outlays by 2007: The Global Fund to Fight AIDS, Tuberculosis, and Malaria (GFATM), $8 billion; and the Global Health Research Fund (GHRF), $1.5 billion. Additional R&D outlays of $1.5 billion per year should be channeled through existing institutions such as TDR, IVR, and HRP at WHO, as well as the Global Forum for Health Research and various public-private partnerships that are currently aiming toward new drug and vaccine development. Country programs should also direct at least 5 percent of outlays to operational research.

5. The supply of other Global Public Goods (GPGs) should be bolstered through additional financing of relevant international agencies such as the World Health Organization and World Bank by $1 billion per year as of 2007 and $2 billion per year as of 2015. These GPGs include disease surveillance at the international level, data collection and analysis of global health trends (such as burden of disease), analysis and dissemination of international best practices in disease control and health systems, and technical assistance and training.

6. To support private-sector incentives for late-stage drug development, existing "orphan drug legislation" in the high-income countries should be modified to cover diseases of the poor such as the tropical vector-borne diseases. In addition, the GFATM and other donor purchasing entities should establish pre-commitments to purchase new targeted products at commercially viable prices.

7. The international pharmaceutical industry, in cooperation with low-income countries and the WHO, should ensure access of the low-income countries to essential medicines through commitments to provide essential medicines at the lowest viable commercial price in the low-income countries, and to license the production of essential medicines to generics producers as warranted by cost and/or supply conditions, as discussed in detail in the Report.

8. The WTO member governments should ensure sufficient safeguards for the developing countries, and in particular the right of countries that do not produce the relevant pharmaceutical products to invoke compulsory licensing for imports from third-country generics suppliers.

9. The International Monetary Fund and World Bank should work with recipient countries to incorporate the scaling up of health and other poverty-reduction programs into a viable macroeconomic framework.

Table 4. RECOMMENDED DONOR AND COUNTRY COMMITMENTS
(billions of constant 2002 US dollars)

	2001 (CMH estimates)	2007	2015
DONOR COMMITMENTS			
Country-level programs:			
Least-Developed Countries	$1.5	$14	$21
Other-Low-Income Countries	$2.0	$6	$8
Middle-Income Countries	$1.5 ODA 0.5 Nonconcessional	$2	$2
of which: Global Fund to Fight AIDS, Tuberculosis, and Malaria	$0	$8	$12
Global Public Goods			
R&D	(<) $0.5	$3	$4
of which: Global Health Research Fund	0	$1.5	$2.5
International Agencies	$1	$2	$3
Total Donor Commitments	$7	$27	$38
DOMESTIC RESOURCES FOR HEALTH			
Least-Developed Countries	$7	$11	$16
Other Low-Income Countries	$43	$62	$74
COUNTRY-LEVEL PROGRAMS IN LOW-INCOME COUNTRIES			
Donor Commitments plus Domestic Resources	$53.5	$93	$119

Note: Recommendations are for annual commitments in a global scaled up program. As stressed throughout the Report, actual disbursements will depend on policy performance within recipient countries.

THE COMMISSION REPORT

The world community has within its power the capacity to save the lives of millions of people every year and to bolster economic development in the world's poorest countries. This Report describes a strategy for achieving those goals by expanding investments in the health of the world's poor. Our conclusions are substantiated by extensive research and consultations undertaken during the past 2 years, especially by the work of six Working Groups, which in total produced 87 background studies and six synthesis monographs to be published by the World Health Organization.[27] The hundreds of participants that joined in this analytical process are listed in Appendix 1 of this Report.

EVIDENCE ON HEALTH AND DEVELOPMENT

The importance of health in its own right cannot be overstressed. In the words of Nobel Laureate Amartya Sen, health (like education) is among the basic capabilities that gives value to human life.[28] In a global survey commissioned for the Millennium Summit of the United Nations by UN Secretary General Kofi Annan (Millennium Poll, United Nations 2000), good health consistently ranked as the number one desire of men and women around the world. The anguish of disease and premature death makes disease control a central preoccupation of all societies, and motivates the inclusion of health among the basic human rights enshrined in international law.[29] The wisdom of every culture also teaches that "health is wealth" in a more instrumental sense as well.[30] For individuals and families, health brings the capacity for personal development and economic security in the future. Health is the basis for job productivity, the capacity to learn in school, and the capability to grow intellectually, physically, and emotionally. In economic terms, health and education are the two cornerstones of human capital, which Nobel Laureates Theodore Shultz and Gary Becker have demonstrated to be the basis of an individual's economic productivity. As with the economic well-being of individual households, good population health is a critical input into poverty reduction, economic growth, and long-term economic development at the scale of whole societies.[31] This point is widely acknowledged by analysts and policy makers, but is greatly underestimated in its qualitative and quantitative significance, and in the investment allocations of many developing-country and donor governments.[32] Societies with a heavy burden of disease tend to experience a multiplicity of severe impediments to economic progress. Conversely, several of the great "takeoffs" in economic history—such as the rapid growth of Britain during the Industrial Revolution; the takeoff of the US South in the early 20th century; the rapid growth of Japan in the early 20th century; and the dynamic development of southern Europe and East Asia beginning in the 1950s and 1960s—were supported by important breakthroughs in public health, disease control, and improved nutritional intake (which, in addition to improving energy levels and productivity of workers, also reduced the vulnerability to infectious disease). The most impressive account of these historical trends comes from the work of Professor Robert Fogel, whose seminal studies have elucidated the relationship between body size and food supply and shown it to be critical for long-term labor productivity (Fogel 1991; 1997; 2000). The secular declines in mortality that have been observed over the past 200 years in Europe have been importantly boosted by the increased availability of calories in the diet, as well as by advances in public health and medical technologies. Fogel states "The increase in the amount of calories available for work over the past 200 years must have made a nontrivial contribution to the growth rate of the per capita income of countries such as France and Great Britain."[33]

The economic costs of avoidable disease, when taken together, are staggeringly high. Disease reduces annual incomes of society, the lifetime incomes of individuals, and prospects for economic growth. The losses are dozens of percent of GNP of the poorest countries each year, which translates into hundreds of billions of US dollars. The Commission found that within the developing countries, the communicable diseases, maternal mortality, and undernutrition hit the poor much harder than they hit the rich, though all income classes are affected. A substantial amount of research at the World Bank (Gwatkin 2000; Gwatkin et al. 2001) documents the vast divide in health status of the relatively high- and low-income groups within a society. For example, mortality rates among the poorest quintile of children in Bolivia and Turkey were found to be as much as four times higher than among the richest quintile.[34] Many other indicators of health outcomes and access to health services showed similar gaps around the world. Moreover, an episode of illness may reduce a poor household to penury, especially when they have to sell their productive assets in order to cover health care outlays. A concerted attack against these diseases, therefore, inherently constitutes a poverty-reduction effort in which the benefits will accrue disproportionately to the poor. Investments in health therefore merit a special pride of place within the strategies for poverty reduction now underway in many low-income countries.

There are many reasons for the increased burden of disease on the poor. First, the poor are much more susceptible to disease because of lack of access to clean water and sanitation, safe housing, medical care, information about preventative behaviors, and adequate nutrition. Second, the poor are much less likely to seek medical care even when it is urgently needed, because of their greater distance from health providers, their lack of out-of-pocket resources needed to cover health outlays, and their lack of knowledge of how best to respond to an episode of illness. Third, as mentioned, out-of-pocket outlays for serious illness can push them into a poverty trap from which they do not recover, by forcing them into debt or into the sale or mortgaging of productive assets (such as land). A serious illness may plunge a household into prolonged impoverishment, extending even to the next generation as children are forced from school and into the workforce.

The macroeconomic evidence confirms that countries with the weakest conditions of health and education have a much harder time achieving sustained growth than do countries with better conditions of health and education. In Table 5, we show the growth rates of several dozen developing countries during the period 1965 to 1994, grouping the countries according to their initial income levels in 1965 and their rates of infant mortality in the same year (as a proxy for overall disease conditions). The

Table 5. GROWTH RATE OF PER CAPITA INCOME, 1965–1994 (according to income and infant mortality rate, 1965)

Initial Infant Mortality Rate, 1965	IMR ≤ 50	50 < IMR ≤ 100	100 < IMR ≤ 150	IMR > 150
Initial Income, 1965 (PPP-adjusted 1990 US dollars)				
GDP ≤$750	—	3.7	1.0	0.1
$750 < GDP ≤ $1,500	—	3.4	1.1	−0.7
$1,500 < GDP ≤ $3,000	5.9	1.8	1.1	2.5
$3,000 < GDP ≤ $6,000	2.8	1.7	0.3	—
GDP > $6,000	1.9	−0.5	—	—

Note: The reported growth rate is the simple average of the GDP growth rates of all countries in the specific cell.

table shows that for any given initial income interval, countries with lower infant mortality rates experienced higher economic growth during the period. For example, in the poorest grouping (less than $750 per person per year in purchasing-power-parity-adjusted 1990 US dollars), countries with an infant mortality rate (IMR) between 50 and 100 per 1,000 live births enjoyed annual average growth of 3.7 percent per year, whereas similarly poor countries with an IMR greater than 150 had average growth of only 0.1 percent per year.[35]

The correlation between better health and higher economic growth holds up even when additional economic variables are introduced to try to account for the cross-country patterns of growth (as in the work of Barro and Sala-i-Martin 1995; Bloom and Sachs 1998; Bhargava et al. 2001). Standard macroeconomic analyses of cross-country growth are based on a model in which economic growth during an interval of time is a function of initial income (because of conditional convergence), economic policy variables, and other structural characteristics of the economy, including indicators of population health. A typical statistical estimate suggests that each 10 percent improvement in life expectancy at birth (LEB) is associated with a rise in economic growth of at least 0.3 to 0.4 percentage points per year, holding other growth factors constant. The difference in annual growth, therefore, accounted for by LEB between a typical high-income country (LEB = 77 years) and a typical least-developed country (LEB = 49 years) is about 1.6 percentage points per year, which cumulates to enormous effects over time.[36] In short, health status seems to explain an important part of the difference in economic growth rates, even after controlling for standard macroeconomic variables. In today's world, poor health has particularly pernicious effects on economic development in sub-Saharan Africa, South Asia, and pockets of high disease and intense poverty elsewhere. Sub-Saharan Africa has experienced a chronic decline of living standards during the past generation, starting from the lowest base in the world. The heavy burden of disease, and its multiple effects on productivity, demography, and education, have certainly played a role in Africa's chronic poor performance. A recent econometric study (Bloom and Sachs 1998) found that more than half of Africa's growth shortfall relative to the high-growth countries of East Asia could be explained statistically by disease burden, demography, and geography, rather than by more traditional variables of macroeconomic policy and political governance. High prevalence of diseases such as malaria and HIV/AIDS are associated with persistent and large reductions of economic growth rates.

High malaria prevalence, for example, has been shown to be associated with a reduction of economic growth of 1 percent per year or more.[37]

The gains in growth of per capita income as a result of improved health are impressive, but tell only a part of the story. Even if per capita economic growth were unaffected by health, there would still be important gains in economic well-being from increased longevity. When comparing well-being across societies, it is important to take account of life expectancy as well as annual income. In healthier countries, individuals live much longer on average, so their lifetime economic earnings are therefore much higher. Consider, for example, the differences in well-being between an average resident of Botswana and of the United States. In Botswana, the reported average annual income in 1997 was about $6,320 in purchasing power adjusted terms.[38] In the United States, the average income the same year was $30,000. At first glance, it would seem that the US income was 5 times higher per person. But an average 22-year-old in Botswana with 12 years of education has a lifetime expected income around 61 times the annual average ($385,000), whereas a similarly educated 22-year-old American, because of a longer expected life span, has a lifetime expected income of around 120 times the annual average ($3,600,000). Thus, in terms of (undiscounted) lifetime incomes rather than annual incomes, the income gap is actually closer to 10 times. The gap in psychological well-being ("utility" in the economist's jargon) would be even larger. Moreover, increased longevity has indirect impacts on economic well-being in addition to the direct effects of more years of earning power, consumption, and leisure. Longer-lived households will tend to invest a higher fraction of their incomes in education and financial saving, because their longer time horizon allows them more years to reap the benefits of such investments.

Because disease weighs so heavily on economic development, investing in health is an important component of an overall development strategy. This is especially true in poor countries where the burden of disease is very high. But investments in health work best as part of a sound overall development strategy. Economic growth requires not only healthy individuals but also education, and other complementary investments, an appropriate division of labor between the public and private sectors, well-functioning markets, good governance, and institutional arrangements that foster technological advance. Private sector–led growth in the business sector must be complemented by an active role of government in several areas: ensuring core investments in health and education, guaranteeing the rule of law, protecting the physical environment, and working in cooperation with the private sector to foster scientific and technological advance. We are not claiming that investments in health can solve development problems, but rather that investments in health should be a central part of an overall development and poverty reduction strategy.

We illustrate the position of health among the many contributors to economic development in Figure 1. Economic output is shown to be a function of policies and institutions (economic policies, governance, and supply of public goods) on the one hand, and factor inputs (human capital, technology, and enterprise capital) on the other. Good policies and institutions are critically important: they help to determine both economic performance for any given levels of capital and technology, and also the pace at which capital and technology accumulate. Health has its most important economic effects on human capital and on enterprise capital, as

Figure 1. HEALTH AS AN INPUT INTO ECONOMIC DEVELOPMENT

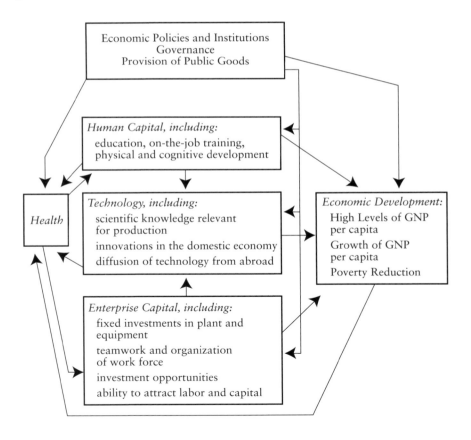

we discuss in the Report, through a variety of pathways—some obvious and others more subtle. Health itself is affected by the prevailing policies and institutions, the level of human capital (since education, for example, promotes health), the level of technology in the society, especially in the health sector itself, and on the very growth in income and poverty reduction that better health engenders.

Economic development is therefore a multi-sectoral process, and the strategy for economic development must build on a broad range of social investments as well as strategies to encourage private-sector business investment. For low-income countries, the emerging PRSP process provides a promising mechanism for incorporating the fight against disease into a more comprehensive development strategy. The PRSP process impels governments and civil society to look across a range of policies in health, education, water and sanitation, environmental management, gender relations, and other areas. We applaud this comprehensive approach, since even on the narrow question of health it is clear that good health and the protection against disease cannot be produced by the health sector alone. One of the most powerful contributors to reduced child mortality, for example, is the literacy of mothers, which is itself the product of an education system that ensures widespread access to education for the poor, including girls as well as boys. Safe water and sanitation, backed by proper hygienic behavior such as hand washing and the use of soap, could dramatically reduce the incidence of many diarrheal and other diseases that kill millions of children each year. And dietary intake interacts critically with disease. Insufficient intake of total calories and proteins, often the result of very low food productivity of peasant farm households, can leave individuals immunosuppressed, making them vastly more vulnerable to the onset and consequences of infectious disease. Micronutrient deficiencies can have devastating consequences for physical and cognitive development. Cultural norms, especially inequalities in relations between men and women, can exacerbate disease conditions. A young girl's vulnerability to AIDS may be little reduced through education about safe sexual practices if the girl remains vulnerable to demands for sexual favors in lopsided relationships with socially powerful men. For all of these reasons, improvements in health should be considered within a comprehensive poverty reduction framework.

Global commitments to improved health are featured in the Millennium Development Goals (MDGs) agreed by the world's heads of government at the Millennium Summit in 2000.[39] The MDGs focus on poverty reduction in general and on several health goals in particular, thereby rightly underscoring the linkages between overall poverty alleviation and investments in health.[40] The MDG health targets include: (1) a reduction in child mortality by two-thirds of the 1990 level by 2015; (2) a reduction in maternal mortality ratios by three-fourths of the 1990 level by 2015; and (3) the end of rising HIV/AIDS and other major disease prevalence no later than 2015. Other recent international initiatives, such as the Roll Back Malaria and Stop TB programs, have added additional and more tightly specified targets for disease control in specific areas.[41]

The MDGs are partly an expression of humanitarian concern, but they are also an investment in the well-being of the rich countries as well as the poor. The evidence is stark: disease breeds instability in poor countries, which rebounds on the rich countries as well. A high infant mortality rate was recently found to be one of the main predictors of subsequent state collapse (through coups, civil war, and other unconstitutional changes in regime) in a study of state failure over the period 1960 to 1994.[42] The United States ended up intervening militarily in many of those crises.[43] In line with this thinking, intelligence studies have stressed the strategic significance of controlling worldwide infectious diseases, including AIDS.[44] Of course, the spillovers are even more than social and political instability in disease-impacted countries: communicable disease in one locale can rapidly spread across international boundaries. AIDS itself is the most dramatic example of a disease that originated in one location and that quickly crossed national and continental boundaries to spread to the rest of the world. The current best guess is that AIDS originated in western Africa around 1931, plus or minus 15 years.[45] An influenza outbreak of a newly mutated strain could be the next example of a worldwide killer, where early detection and case management could save a huge number of lives in rich and poor countries alike.[46] Multi-drug resistant tuberculosis (MDR-TB) is similarly crossing borders from poor to rich countries.[47]

Within societies, diseases that afflict the poor adversely affect the rich as well—through the spread of infections and the broader destabilization of society. A striking example involves the effectiveness of insecticide-treated mosquito nets (ITNs) in the control of malaria. Experimental data show that the effectiveness of ITNs is enhanced by a high level of utilization of ITNs within a village, so that an individual bednet user is more protected if others are also using nets.[48] This is because ITNs work not only by stopping the bites of mosquitoes through the net, but also (or even mainly) by reducing the subsequent infectivity of mosquitoes that come into contact with the insecticide on the net, thereby reducing the incidence of malaria through the village. An ITN user may still get bitten, but the biting mosquito is much less likely to be infective if others in the village are also using ITNs. Thus, the rich members of a village have a direct stake in the use of ITNs by the poor households as well. Similar examples of such "spillovers" or "mass effects" abound in infectious disease control. For example, untreated cases of TB among the poor are likely to spread, and poorly treated cases are likely to develop multi-drug resistant TB, with dire consequences for the rest of society.

A final example: the higher is the proportion of immunization coverage in the society, the higher is the probability that the nonimmunized will be protected as well from epidemic transmission of the disease, a phenomenon known as *herd immunity*. The positive spillovers of immunization are clearest in the case of complete eradication of a disease, such as the triumph over smallpox. Today the world saves hundreds of millions of dollars each year on routine smallpox immunization programs, which are no longer necessary now that the disease has been eradicated. To achieve these savings, every case of smallpox had to be eliminated, which in turn depended on mass immunization of the poorest of the poor, which in turn required investments by the richer countries. The evidence developed by the Commission, consistent with many other studies, suggests that that the Millennium Development Goals for poverty reduction and health will not be met without a concerted effort aimed at extending health interventions to the world's poor. Dozens of countries are off track now regarding child mortality, maternal mortality, and curbing the major epidemic diseases. According to the United Nations Development Program (2001), 62 percent of the population of developing countries are in nations that are "lagging, far behind, or slipping" in meeting the infant and child mortality goals.[49] Health systems in poor countries are not yet up to the task of meeting the MDGs, and donor support remains grossly insufficient. The world has made solemn pledges to address the crises of disease of the poor, but has not yet taken strong enough practical steps to implement them. With millions dying unnecessary and tragic deaths, and with global institutions under stress, a scaled-up war against disease is vital for the legitimacy of globalization.

CHANNELS OF INFLUENCE FROM DISEASE TO ECONOMIC DEVELOPMENT

There are three main ways that disease impedes economic well-being and development.[50] The first channel already noted is the most direct: avoidable disease reduces the number of years of healthy life expectancy. The economic losses to society of truncated lives—due to the combination of early deaths and chronic disability—are phenomenally large: hundreds of billions of US dollars per year, representing a significant percentage of the national incomes of the low-income countries. As a result of the AIDS pandemic alone, aggregate economic growth will slow several percentage points per year in Africa, as individuals in the prime of their working lives are struck down. The second channel is the effect of disease on parental investments in children. Societies with high rates of infant mortality (deaths under 1 year of age) and child mortality (deaths under 5 years of age) have higher rates of fertility, in part to compensate for the frequent deaths of children. Large numbers of children, in turn, reduce the ability of poor families to invest heavily in the health and education of each child, a process described by Gary Becker and colleagues as the "quality-quantity tradeoff" in child rearing. The third channel is the depressing effects of disease on the returns to business and infrastructure investment, beyond the effects on individual worker productivity. Whole industries, in agriculture, mining, manufacturing, and tourism, as well as important infrastructure projects, are undermined by a high prevalence of disease. In addition, epidemic and endemic diseases can also undermine social cooperation and even political and macroeconomic stability.

Direct Loss of Well-Being to the Individual

Individuals lose economic well-being as a result of disease. When economists and public health specialists try to account quantitatively for that loss of well-being, they usually divide it into three parts: (1) the reduction in market income caused by disease; (2) the reduction in longevity caused by disease; and (3) the reduction in psychological well-being caused by disease, often labeled "pain and suffering," even when there is no reduction in market income or longevity.[51] The reduction in market income, in turn, has at least four sub-components: (i) the costs of medical treatment; (ii) the loss of labor-market income from a episode of illness; (iii) the loss of adult earning power from episodes of disease in childhood; and (iv) the loss of future earnings from premature mortality.

One goal of economic analysis is to convert these disease-induced losses into dollar terms, in order to assess the economic benefits that would accrue to reducing the disease burden. The economics literature on the value of life has a very strong and consistent conclusion: the value of an extra year of healthy life—as a result of successfully treating a disease, for example—is worth considerably more than the extra market income that will be earned in the year. According to some estimates, each life year is valued at around three times the annual earnings. This multiple of earnings reflects the value of leisure time in addition to market consumption, the pure longevity effect, and the pain and suffering associated with disease. When an individual dies young, the economic losses are calculated as the summation of losses associated with each year of lost life. According to such calculations, a lost life at age 20 is sometimes taken to be equal to 100 times or more the annual earnings, since 40 or more years are lost, and each lost year is worth about three times the annual earnings. Such high valuations have been used in several recent economic analyses.[52]

Whatever the precise numbers, the calculations remind us of something important. When we assess the costs of a disease on society, we must ask not only how the disease affects the level and growth of per capita GNP (for example by reducing worker productivity), but also how the disease affects the lifespan and lifetime earnings lost by society. Even if the AIDS pandemic has no effect on per capita GNP, its effect of reducing longevity would still be devastating to economic well-being. With the average life span in hard-hit countries cut short by years or decades, AIDS is reducing lifetime earnings and economic well-being by a substantial magnitude.

Let us illustrate the enormous costs of malaria and AIDS on African well-being by using these concepts. We multiply the annual number of lost life years due to each disease by some multiple of per capita income to get a rough estimate of the aggregate economic loss. In sub-Saharan Africa, for example, malaria accounted for an estimated 36 million disability adjusted life years (DALYs) lost in 1999 out of a population of 616 million. If each DALY is valued very conservatively as equal to per capita income, the total cost of malaria would be valued at 5.8 percent (= 36 / 616) of the gross national product of the region. If instead we value each DALY at three times the per capita income, the total cost would be 17.4 percent of GNP (= 5.8 percent × 3). Similarly, given an estimate of 72 million DALYs due to AIDS, and assuming each DALY is valued at the per capita income, the economic value of lost life years in 1999 due to AIDS would be 11.7 percent (= 72 / 616) of the gross national product of sub-Saharan Africa. If instead we value each DALY at three times the per capita income, the losses are an astounding 35.1 percent of GNP. Note that each AIDS death is estimated to have resulted in 34.6 DALYs lost on average in 1999.[53] This is because AIDS deaths tend to occur in young adults, so that each death is associated with many life years lost between the age of death and the benchmark of life expectancy.

Note that these cost estimates do not include the effects of disease on the level of annual per capita income itself. Econometric estimates suggest that in the short term, an economy in which the population is at zero risk of malaria tends to grow more than 1 percentage point per year more rapidly than an economy with high malaria risk, controlling for other determinants of growth (such as income level, schooling, quality of institutions, and fiscal policy). Since that growth effect cumulates over time, the econometric estimates suggest that the malarious economy ends up with a per capita income that is roughly half the per capita income of the non-malarious economy, again holding constant the other determinants of growth.[54] These effects on the level of per capita income can be combined with the shorter life span due to malaria to give the overall effect of the disease, which is clearly dozens of percent of GNP lost due to malaria. Even if the precise estimates are open to considerable uncertainty, the magnitude of the economic losses is clear.

The economic consequences of a disease episode on an individual household can be magnified if the cost of dealing with the illness forces a household to spend so much of its resources on medical care that it depletes its assets and debts are incurred. This may throw a household into poverty from which it cannot escape, and which has ramifications for the welfare of all its members and often of relatives as well. The Commission reviewed many studies showing how poor households are rarely insured against catastrophic illness, and are therefore often required to sell their few assets, such as farm implements and animals, or to mortgage their land, in order to maintain minimal consumption in the face of lost market earnings and to pay for urgent medical care. This depletion of productive assets can lead to a poverty trap (ie, persisting poverty) at the household level even after the acute illness is overcome, since impoverished households will have a hard time re-capitalizing their productive activities. The indebted household will lack the working capital to make the short-term investments (e.g., in seed, fertilizer) to produce sufficient output to pay off the debts, and will be unable to borrow against future earnings. The poverty in turn may intensify the original disease conditions as well.[55]

Life Cycle Consequences

Although most studies of the economic burden of disease look only at the costs associated directly with an episode of illness (and with premature mortality when applicable), nonfatal disease episodes early in life can have adverse effects over the entire life cycle. Disease in infancy and in utero can be associated with lifetime sequelae, including both cognitive and physical infirmities.[56] Education is widely recognized as a key to economic development, but many fail to appreciate how important childhood health is for educational attainment. Poor health directly reduces cognitive potential and indirectly undermines schooling through absenteeism, insufficient attention to lessons, and early dropouts.

The long-term consequences of early disease episodes are poorly elucidated but large. Some of the channels are biological: early disease impedes physical and cognitive development, which in turn reduces adult economic productivity. Some are economic as well, as when reduced cognitive capacity leads to premature school leaving, so that the individual carries a lifetime dual burden of reduced cognitive capacity compounded by a lack of educational attainment. Some ingenious indirect evidence suggests that the economic fallout from childhood disease and dietary insufficiency is enormous, much larger than typically believed. In many developing countries that have been studied, adult height is strongly and positively correlated with adult earnings (shown in Figure 2 in the case of

Figure 2. BRAZIL: HEIGHT AND WAGES

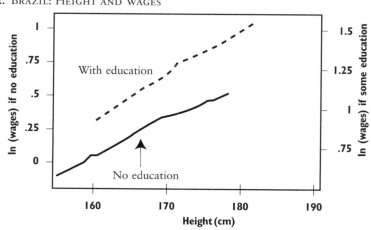

Source: Strauss and Thomas, 1998.

Brazil). Adult height is itself a reflection of childhood nutrition and disease experience. Children that suffer repeated bouts of infectious disease and that receive insufficient nutrition in the diet are likely to reach adulthood with reduced height. The correlation of height and earnings is therefore a surprisingly strong indication of how childhood experience in health and nutrition has lifetime consequences in economic productivity.

One of the most important effects of ill health is to hinder educational attainment, both through effects on cognitive ability and effects on school attendance. Balasz et al. (1986) and Pollitt (1997; 2001) have reviewed the studies that link nutrition and brain development in children. In most of these studies, deficits in key nutrients (iron, vitamin A) are associated with deficits of cognitive ability. Similarly, Bhargava (1997) analyzed a comprehensive longitudinal survey of Tanzanian schoolchildren and found that the health and nutritional status were important predictors of cognitive and educational achievement test results. He also concluded that the removal of intestinal parasites such as hookworm and schistosomiasis is important for child development. An experimental study by Kremer and Miguel (1999) reached a similar conclusion regarded deworming. In a randomized study of treatment of schoolchildren against hookworm, roundworm, and schistosomiasis, children in the treated schools demonstrated significantly higher attendance rates than children in schools without treatment programs. Interestingly, higher attendance was noted for untreated children within the treated schools, suggesting a spillover effect of school attendance from the treated children to the untreated children (e.g., through social norms).

The cost-of-illness literature probably dramatically understates the costs of nonfatal chronic conditions at all stages of the life cycle. Healthier workers are physically and mentally more energetic and robust, more productive, and earn higher wages. Their productivity makes companies more profitable, and a healthy workforce is important when attracting foreign direct investment. They are also less likely to be absent from work due to illness (or illness in their family) and to be more productive on the job. The effect is especially strong in developing countries, where a higher proportion of the workforce is engaged in manual labor. In Indonesia, for example, anemic men were found to be 20 percent less productive than men who were not. When the anemic men were treated with iron, their productivity increased nearly to the levels of the non-anemic men.[57] There is also the relationship between early health and success in education mentioned in the preceding paragraph. Healthy children are able to learn better and become better-educated (and higher earning) adults. In a healthy family, children's education is less likely to be interrupted due to their ill health or the ill health of their family. The importance of hookworm is shown in another one of the more classical examples of ill health interfering with productive activity. Much of the early economic development of the Southern United States has been linked to the elimination of hookworm and its attendant anemia. Ettling (1981) describes lucidly the effects and conquest of the "germ of laziness" that was responsible for low productive capacity.

Intergenerational Spillovers of Disease
Disease of one individual within the family may have important adverse consequences for other family members, especially the children. An adult's illness may result in poor health, or even death, of a previously healthy child because of a drop off in care giving and family income. The parent's illness or death may force a child to leave school prematurely, for example, in order to help support the family. The adult's illness will also reduce the transfer of knowledge from parent to child. AIDS-impacted communities in Africa are reporting that the orphaned children are now growing up without the knowledge of local farming.

One the most pernicious, and least recognized, costs of high rates of infant mortality and child mortality works through demography. Poor families compensate for children's deaths by having a large number of children. The logic is painfully clear. Parents may choose to have as many as six or more children just to assure themselves of a high probability that at least one son (or daughter, or both) will survive till the parents' old age. Yet when poor families have so many children, as in much of Africa today, the household can afford only a very small investment in the education and health of each child. Thus, a high burden of disease translates into large families with a low investment per child in education and health. Although high mortality rates of children are by no means the only reasons for high fertility rates (gender inequalities, lack of mothers' education and opportunities for work, and cultural norms being some other factors), a reduction in mortality rates can be a big spur to reduced fertility when combined with family planning, education, and greater labor force participation of women.

The evidence linking fertility levels to infant (under age 1) and child (under age 5) mortality rates is powerful. Figure 3 is a scatterplot for 148 countries in 1995 showing the striking correlation of the total fertility rate

Figure 3. RELATIONSHIP OF INFANT MORTALITY RATE (X-AXIS) AND TOTAL FERTILITY
RATE (Y-AXIS), 148 COUNTRIES, 1995 (partial-regression plot)

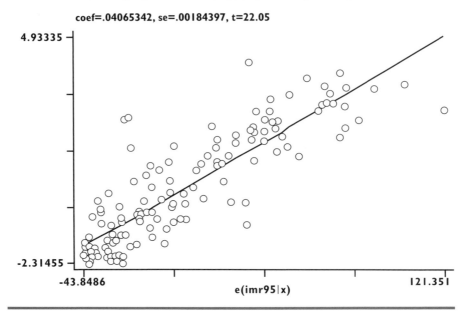

(TFR, y-axis) and the infant mortality rate (IMR, x-axis).[58] Countries with
an IMR of less than 20 have an average TFR of 1.7 children. Countries
with an IMR of over 100 have an average TFR of 6.2 children. The probability of childhood survival is not the only factor in the transition from
high to low fertility, but it is an important one. The mother's education is
certainly another factor. More educated mothers not only have greater
control over the reproductive choices within the household, but they also
have a higher earning power in the marketplace, and therefore a greater
opportunity cost to staying home to raise children. The availability of
family planning services, including access to contraception and family
counseling, is also another important factor. Cultural norms are also critical, as is migration to urban areas.[59]

It is ironic that high mortality rates of children tend to provoke high
fertility rates among poor couples. In general, the high fertility more than
compensates for the high mortality, an implication of risk aversion of
households. In one numerical illustration, households whose children have
a 75-percent survival rate choose to have six children, of whom an average of 4.5 survive. The households whose children have a 95-percent survival rate have two children, of whom an average of 1.9 survive. The high-

Figure 4. RELATIONSHIP OF LOG (INFANT MORTALITY RATE) AND POPULATION GROWTH RATE, 148 COUNTRIES, 1995 (partial-regression plot)

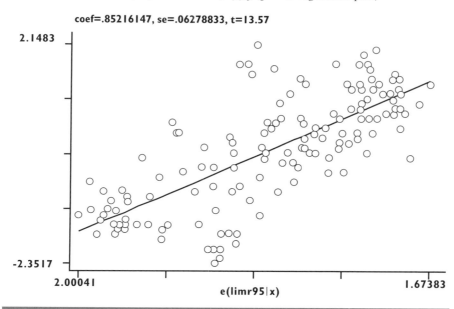

coef=.85216147, se=.06278833, t=13.57

mortality households end up with a higher population growth rate than the low-mortality households, perhaps counterintuitively. But this pattern helps us to understand the surprising fact that countries with high infant mortality rates have the fastest growing populations in the world, with consequent strains on the physical environment, especially to the extent that increasing populations are crowding fragile subsistence farm lands. The strong positive correlation between the infant mortality rate and the overall population growth rate is shown in Figure 4. Lowering infant mortality rates will tend to lower, not raise, population growth rate over the longer run. As noted earlier, however, disease control programs should be complemented by reproductive health and education programs to ensure that the transition to lower mortality is accompanied as rapidly as possible by the transition to lower fertility.

Demographic effects operate not just at the household (micro) level but at the economy-wide (macro) level. When child mortality rates decline, followed by declines in fertility rates, overall population growth tends to slow and the average age of the population tends to rise. The youth-dependency ratio (number of youths per number of adults) also tends to decline. These demographic changes boost overall per capita GNP and economic growth (see Bloom and Canning 2001). The rising proportion of the population at working age directly raises GNP per capita.[60] The share of the population at ages with high saving rates increases, so that aggregate saving rates in the economy tend to rise. The longer life expectancy of each individual also tends to raise the age-adjusted saving rates as well. These effects, like others that we are examining, are evident in the cross-country savings patterns, though the magnitudes of effects are hard to estimate with precision, given the number of confounding variables.

Disease and Societal Spillovers

Diseases impose costs on society beyond the costs to individuals and families specifically affected by disease episodes. A high disease burden, for example, creates a high turnover of the labor force and lowers the profitability of enterprises beyond any direct effects on individual worker productivity.[61] Diseases such as malaria pose risks to all individuals who may enter a particular location, and therefore depress tourism, block otherwise profitable investments, or prevent the effective economic use of arable land or other natural resources. Many other tropical parasitic diseases (e.g., onchocerciasis, schistosomiasis, and trypanosomiasis) similarly render certain tropical areas unlivable or extremely unattractive for certain forms of settlement or agriculture. A high incidence of disease among a firm's labor force also causes very high turnover and absenteeism, which depresses profits beyond the effects of individual disease episodes. On average, firms must hire and train more than one worker for each position to compensate for high turnover. Many firms have reportedly cut back on investments in southern Africa because of the high prevalence of AIDS, which leads to expectations of very high worker turnover.

The classic example of disease impeding a critical investment is the construction of the Panama Canal. It is estimated that ten to twenty thousand people died primarily from malaria and yellow fever in the first years of the project between 1882 and 1888, and this was perhaps the dominant reason for the failure of de Lesseps to repeat the triumph of Suez in the Americas. The cost of the failure was about 30 million dollars and decades of delay in completing the Canal. The experience gained by William Gorgas in controlling those diseases in Havana, which was applied in Panama, was one of the main factors that led to the successful completion of the canal by the United States in 1914 (Jones 1990). Similar problems in controlling diseases today continue to plague investments in mining, tourism, and agriculture. Circumstantial evidence suggests that the dramatic reduction of malaria in several subtropical regions in the 1940s and 1950s (notably the southern European countries of Greece, Italy, Portugal, and Spain) had a galvanizing effect on economic growth to a large extent by spurring massive tourism and foreign direct investment.[62] Such gains would greatly exceed the direct costs of the disease as would have been measured in a cost of illness study.

The risks to enterprises of AIDS in southern Africa seem similarly to be taking an enormous toll on investments in the region. Part of an enterprise's productivity results from the teamwork that is engendered by stable working relations among key personnel. With the massive turnover resulting from AIDS, firms are constantly facing the rupturing of work groups and the heavy costs of re-assigning and re-training workers. Such turnover costs are a direct burden to enterprise profitability, costs that are additional to the effects on individual worker productivity. The *Economist*, for example, reports examples of multinationals in South Africa hiring three workers for each skilled position "to ensure that replacements are on hand when trained workers die."[63] There is considerable anecdotal evidence of enterprises cutting back their investments in southern Africa as a result of AIDS.

In a similar vein, when a significant proportion of individuals in a community get sick, the entire community suffers through spillover effects. The local budget may shift to care for the ill, thereby reducing money available for other social services. The level of trust in the community may fall, especially if the disease is interpreted as a curse, or as poisoning, or as case of witchcraft, as frequently reported in parts of Africa in response to AIDS. Skilled workers may flee or die, leaving the community without the technical or entrepreneurial leadership that it requires. Social morale may flag. Large numbers of orphans left by AIDS may strain the social support networks. Household saving rates are likely to fall, and with that the rate of society-wide capital accumulation. Even the direct time and expense of the frequent vigils and funerals may have a significant adverse effect on the local economy, a phenomenon clearly apparent in some of the southern African countries heavily affected by HIV/AIDS.

A high disease burden disrupts the national budget just as it disrupts a family's budget. The health care system is strained, and requires more resources, including perhaps donor resources that might otherwise have gone to meeting other needs. Tax revenues collected by the government are reduced to the extent that economic activity is diminished (such as when tourism declines or enterprise output is disrupted for other reasons). The combination of increased budget demands and reduced budget revenues may lead to significant budget deficits that in turn destabilize the macroeconomy, with further adverse effects on the economy.

THE EPIDEMIOLOGY OF DISEASE IN LOW-INCOME COUNTRIES

The population health of developing countries in recent decades has been a story of good news, bad news, and disastrous news. The good news is that in most regions of the developing world, the second half of the twentieth century saw an unparalleled improvement in global public health. Between 1960 and 1995, life expectancy in the low-income countries of the world improved by 22 years, as opposed to 8 in the developed countries. On a global average, the under-five mortality rate declined from 150 per 1,000 live births in the 1950s to 40 per 1,000 live births in the 1990s, with marked decreases in every decade. These gains, moreover, did not simply occur by themselves, as a natural fallout of economic development. They rather reflect the power of health care and related investments. Over the past three decades, various immunization campaigns and child survival strategies have increased by millions the number of children protected against the predations of common childhood infections. Mortality has also fallen among nonsmoking adults. Both these gains have been aided by other factors, including particularly the spread of education. These gains therefore show the efficacy of well-targeted investments in health, and presage what can now be accomplished.

The bad news is that despite these impressive achievements, the total burden of preventable disease in developing countries remains shockingly high, with profound human and economic costs. As we saw in Table 1, life expectancy in the 48 least-developed countries is just 51 years, compared with 78 in the high-income countries.[64] Infant mortality rates are 100 per 1,000 live births in the least-developed countries, compared with just 6 in the high-income countries. According to WHO estimates for 1998, infectious diseases were the world's biggest killer of children and adults. They accounted for 13.3 million out of a worldwide total of almost 54 million deaths. In 1998, up to 45 percent of deaths in Africa and Southeast Asia are thought to have been due to an infectious disease, while worldwide 48 percent of premature deaths (under age 45) are thought to have had an infectious etiology. For low- and middle-income countries combined, almost a third of deaths were due to preventable and/or treatable conditions of communicable diseases, maternal and perinatal conditions, and

Table 6. AIDS Epidemic, Selected Regions, end-1999 (000s)

Region	People living with HIV/AIDS, end-1999	AIDS Deaths, 1999	AIDS Orphans, 1999	Adult Prevalence (%), end-1999
Global	34,300	2,800	13,200	1.07
Sub-Saharan Africa	24,500	2,200	12,100	8.57
East Asia and Pacific	530	18	5	0.06
South and Southeast Asia	5,600	460	850	0.54
Eastern Europe and Central Asia	420	8	15	0.21
North Africa and Middle East	220	13	15	0.12
Western Europe	520	7	9	0.23
North America	900	20	70	0.58
Caribbean	360	30	85	2.11

Source: UNAIDS, Report on the Global HIV/AIDS Epidemic, *June 2000.*

nutritional deficiencies. The death toll from these diseases in a single year is staggering: 16 million deaths, with just a few conditions causing the lion's share. Effective interventions exist to reduce the mortality associated with each of these conditions, but these interventions do not reach hundreds of millions of people on a reliable basis. If we consider just the case of vaccine-preventable diseases, the Global Alliance on Vaccines and Immunizations (GAVI) estimates that worldwide there are 2.9 million deaths per year from diseases readily combated by immunization, the overwhelming proportion in developing countries.[65]

The disastrous news is that one single new virus, the human immunodeficiency virus (HIV) that causes AIDS, has in just one generation plummeted much of sub-Saharan Africa and some other parts of the world into the most devastating pandemic in modern history. The first cases of HIV were identified in the early 1980s, presumably after the virus crossed over from an animal virus in mutated form into human populations some decades earlier. But in just 20 years, HIV/AIDS has caused an estimated 22 million deaths (including 2.8 million in 1999), brought untold human suffering, and infected a total of 58 million people, of whom 36 million are now alive. (Table 6, with data for the end of 1999, shows 34.3 million people infected.) Most of these individuals are likely to die premature deaths from the complications of AIDS, though their lives may be greatly extended by current treatment protocols, and even saved from AIDS if improved technologies are successfully developed in the coming years. In some societies, particularly in eastern and southern Africa, the pandemic has advanced to an alarming stage in which a quarter or more of the adult population is infected. In many other parts of the world, especially the highly populous regions of Asia, the pandemic is in a early stage, posing threats that tens of millions more will succumb in the coming years unless effective control strategies that have already been identified are introduced on a much wider and more intensive scale.

The health prospects of the poorest billion could be radically improved by targeting a relatively small set of diseases and conditions. The primary targets are:

HIV/AIDS

malaria

tuberculosis

maternal and perinatal conditions

widespread causes of child mortality including measles, tetanus, diphtheria, acute respiratory infection, and diarrheal disease

malnutrition that exacerbates those diseases

other vaccine-preventable illness

tobacco-related disease

These conditions are not the only health problems that afflict the poor: the poor contract everyone else's diseases as well as the diseases heavily concentrated among themselves. However, these diseases account for a large proportion of avoidable mortality of the poor, where we measure avoidable mortality by comparing the death rates in poor countries with the death rates experienced by nonsmokers in the richest countries on an age-adjusted basis.[66] We therefore focus on the conditions associated with the greatest excess mortality in the poor countries relative to the rich countries, and note that these conditions afflict mainly the poor within the low-income countries.

Breaking the results down into three age groups, the study found that avoidable mortality accounts for about 87 percent of the total chance of death among children up to the age of 5 in low- and middle-income countries. Among males aged from 5 to 29, 60 percent of total mortality was calculated to be avoidable, while for females in the same cohort the figure was 82 percent, the higher level largely due to risks incurred through pregnancy and childbirth. Among women from 30 to 69, 51 percent of the mortality was avoidable; only among men in that age range did avoidable mortality fall to less than half total mortality, at 43 percent.

It should be obvious that not all the "avoidable" mortality identified by this approach can, in fact, be avoided in the near term, since to do so would involve immediately raising environments and health systems to the standards of developed countries; though this process need not be as slow as many might imagine and can surely be accelerated, it cannot be rendered arbitrarily short. But it is not unreasonable to think of this level of care as an ultimate aspiration.

ADDRESSING THE DISEASE BURDEN

Crucially, there are already effective interventions that can reduce the mortality associated with each of these diseases, though obviously it is also important that better ways of treating and preventing many of these diseases be developed. Some of these diseases may even be susceptible to elimination; all can be controlled to some extent, and that extent is often large. Progress is limited neither by an intractably large range of options, nor mainly by ignorance of what needs to be done. The usual complex and interlocking problems of poverty are all operative: the poor may lack the knowledge to protect themselves adequately or seek needed services; they may lack the power to protect their rights; or they may lack income to access services. The best way forward is on two tracks. One is investing in the health system—to make it strong enough, and well-funded enough, and with the right priorities to deliver a relatively small number of essential interventions. The other is by complementary steps in education and in broader institutional advances, such as community involvement, so that the poor can effectively get access to and are motivated to seek out these essential interventions.

Striking progress can and has been made in many disease categories and most regions of the world. A particularly conspicuous form of progress has been the historically unprecedented ability to move beyond the control of some diseases to their elimination or eradication.[67] The eradication of smallpox stands with landing on the moon as a paradigm-shift in human achievement. For today's skeptics, it is useful to recall that many believed that smallpox eradication would also be impossible; the vote to pursue smallpox eradication passed the World Health Assembly in 1966 by two votes![68] Polio, already humbled to such an extent that its contribution to the global burden of disease is minimal, is likely to be eradicated in the near future. Such eradications are not merely great public-health achievements: they may also represent a recurrent saving in the form of vaccinations no longer required.[69] Similarly, the elimination of measles, still a major killer—800,000 deaths in 1998—is no longer out-side the bounds of possibility for major regions. Even global eradication may be feasible if global vaccination levels can be raised. Malawi, one of the poorest countries in the world, where 20 percent of the population has no access to health services and less than 50 percent has access to safe water, has recently committed itself to high levels of routine measles immunization and to campaigns to catch those missed out by routine efforts. In 1999, there were no reported children's deaths due to measles in Malawi, and only two confirmed cases were seen throughout the coun-try. In addition to programs aimed at elimination of polio and measles, WHO is currently leading initiatives, greatly supported by donations from the pharmaceutical industry and support from nongovernmental organi-zations, aimed at the global eradication or elimination of seven other dis-eases, most of which impose their heaviest burden on poor communities: Chagas disease, guinea-worm disease, leprosy, lymphatic filariasis, neona-tal tetanus, iodine deficiency disorders, and blinding trachoma.

Vaccination is not the only vehicle for success. Where implemented, directly observed treatment, short-course (DOTS) for tuberculosis is achieving excellent cure rates.[70] For malaria, the introduction of modern insecticides and improved case management (ie, treatments of patients with anti-malarials) can have a significant impact—in much of Asia and Latin America, deaths due to malaria have been reduced spectacularly. The recent resurgence of the disease, while worrying, has never threatened these countries with death tolls like those of the past. In Africa, pilot proj-ects using insecticide-treated mosquito nets have shown high efficacy in reducing mortality rates when there are high levels of mosquito net use. Diarrheal disease can be addressed by widespread promotion of oral rehy-dration therapy, along with improved sanitation. Such interventions have made significant inroads into the dreadful toll of this disease among chil-dren: deaths from diarrheal disease around the world has dropped from 4.6 million a year in 1980 to 3.3 million a year in 1990 to 1.5 million a year in 1999.

Some specific case studies of successes with these diseases have recent-ly been compiled by the lead international agencies involved in health, to stress the actual successes, on the ground, in many countries around the world. [71] These include:

HIV/AIDS

Drop in HIV prevalence in military conscripts in Thailand

Increasing condom use by sex workers and declining STIs
in Thailand

Reduced HIV prevalence among 13- to 19-year-olds in Uganda

TB

Reduction, due to DOTS, of TB cases in Peru

Reduction, due to DOTS, of mortality rate from TB in China, India,
and Nepal

Malaria

Sharp reduction in malaria deaths in Viet Nam due to improved
case management and insecticide-treated mosquito nets

Reduced malaria incidence in Azerbaijan due to insecticide spraying,
chemoprophylaxis, larviciding, and improved case management

Reduced malaria incidence in coastal Kenya due to insecticide-
treated mosquito nets

Childhood Diseases

Reduced child mortality rate in Mexico through oral rehydration
therapy

Reduced deaths from respiratory infection in Pakistan

Dramatic fall, due to immunization, in measles cases and deaths in
Malawi

Reduced severe anemia in the United Republic of Tanzania through
school-based de-worming

Sharp reduction in child mortality rates through community-based
programs in Brazil

Maternal and Perinatal Conditions

Reduction of maternal deaths through skilled birth attendants in
Sri Lanka

Reduction of mother-to-child transmission of HIV through
antiretroviral drugs

Reduction of mother and infant deaths due to immunization with
tetanus toxoid in Bangladesh

Tobacco-Related Illness

Drop in cigarette sales and rise in tax revenues through an increase
in excise taxes on cigarettes in South Africa

Comprehensive bans on tobacco advertising and promotion in
Poland, South Africa, and Thailand

Impressive as they are, though, such achievements represent at best a
half-finished task. Although one must be impressed that the world has
reduced child mortality rates from 150 per thousand to 40 per thousand

live births, one must at the same time realize that in Africa the rate is still 150 per thousand, and that in some African countries, as a result of HIV/AIDS, the rate is rising rather than falling. Ominously, the situation is not just one of incomplete progress, but one of incipient backsliding. Improvements in public health worldwide are slowing down, and are being reversed in regions of high HIV/AIDS prevalence. Although child mortality around the world has declined in every decade since the 1950s, it did so at a significantly higher rate in the 1970s and 1980s than it did in the 1990s.

In some of the world's poorest countries, the coverage of many basic interventions is falling, not rising. In many countries, the percentage of mothers whose births were attended by trained midwives or doctors is falling. Despite the importance of vaccination for child survival, levels of childhood vaccination stagnated or dropped in many poor countries in the 1990s, leaving tens of millions of children uncovered by immunizations. As a result, children in poor countries still suffer 1.6 million deaths every year due to measles, tetanus, and pertussis, even though these diseases have been substantially eliminated in the high-income countries. Improvements in the reach of immunization services could drastically reduce this number, as has been shown in many countries with successful aggressive efforts against measles. Coverage with other valuable and effective vaccines widely used in the developed world is even poorer. Many vaccines in routine use in the rich countries (such as hepatitis B and *Haemophilus influenzae* type b, or Hib) have barely been introduced into some low-income countries. It is estimated that about one-quarter of the 1.8 million children who die of acute lower respiratory tract infection each year succumb to *Haemophilus influenzae* type b and perhaps an equivalent proportion to Streptococcus pneumonia, for which a new vaccine has recently been introduced in high-income countries.

One of the most important health interventions is greater attention to reproductive health, not only to control the spread of sexually transmitted infections (STIs) such as HIV/AIDS, but also to limit fertility through family planning, including access to contraception.[72] Many of the most disease-burdened places on earth have very high population growth rates, putting enormous stress on these societies and their development prospects.[73] While the high-income countries have population growth rates below 1 percent per year (0.7 percent in 1990–1998), the poorest countries have population growth rates of about 2 percent per year (2.0 percent in 1990–1998), or 2.6 percent excluding China and India.

Although we did not ourselves make cost estimates of the increasing need for family planning services and an adequate supply of contraception, there is clearly a donor financing gap here that will have to be addressed, though it represents only a modest proportion of total funding needs.[74]

Many people wonder whether reducing the death rates in the low-income countries wouldn't thereby exacerbate the population pressures, leading the societies to face increased hardships of hunger, land scarcity, and falling output per person. The question is a valid one: if more individuals are saved through health interventions, for what kind of life are they being saved? The answer, fortunately, is an optimistic one. Health interventions, if well managed, will contribute to slower, not faster, population growth, but for this to occur it is important to combine health interventions with intensified efforts to offer family planning services and increased access to contraception. We've already noted that poor households will choose to have fewer children (and to invest more in the education and health of each child) if they are confident that the children will survive and if they have access to family planning and contraception. With effective family planning programs, the lag between falling mortality rates of children and falling birth rates can be cut sharply, or even eliminated. Bangladesh and several states of southern India (especially Tamil Nadu and Andhra Pradesh) are examples of places that eliminated the lag between falling death rates and falling birth rates, thereby enjoying improved health and declining population growth at the same time.[75]

THE AIDS PANDEMIC

Of all the health problems facing the poorest people of the world, the HIV/AIDS pandemic is undoubtedly the most dramatic. The pandemic has reached every country in the world, and in many it is worsening rapidly. In southern and eastern Africa, infection is running at levels unprecedented for any disease so consistently fatal. The damage done already in these countries, and the potential over the coming decade for deaths on a scale not seen in any previous pandemic, make HIV/AIDS a unique challenge to health systems on a global scale. Three million people died of AIDS in 2000, of whom 2.4 million were in sub-Saharan Africa. Twelve million children in Africa have already been orphaned by the disease, and that number could grow to a staggering 40 million by the end of this decade if more effective control measures are not undertaken. The disease will devastate African society and cripple economic development in Africa and other high-prevalence regions unless brought under control.

Although HIV/AIDS is a global problem, the pandemic looks very different in different places. Nearly three-quarters of persons living with HIV/AIDS are in sub-Saharan Africa. In eastern and southern Africa, the disease has spread quickly and widely throughout the population. HIV prevalence in antenatal clinic attendees doubled from 18 percent to 35 percent in Botswana from 1994 to 1999, and in South Africa increased from 3 percent to 20 percent over the same time period. In central and western Africa, from 2 to 10 percent of adults are infected. Heterosexual transmission is the dominant source of new cases in sub-Saharan Africa, and more women than men are infected. An explosive increase in new HIV infections has taken place in the countries of the former Soviet Union, due primarily to transmission by injection drug use. All of the countries with severe AIDS epidemics in South and East Asia, with the exception of Cambodia, have also experienced early and dramatic epidemics among injecting drug users. In addition, Cambodia, India, Myanmar, and Thailand have large epidemics based on heterosexual transmission. The epidemic in the Caribbean is also predominantly heterosexual, with some of the highest infection rates outside of sub-Saharan Africa. Throughout South America, national HIV prevalence is generally 1 percent or less, spread mainly through sex between men and injection drug use. Outside of sub-Saharan Africa, more men than women are living with HIV/AIDS.

The reasons for the variations in prevalence between countries are not entirely clear. The time since the epidemic's introduction is certainly a factor, as are patterns of mobility, sexual activity, and perhaps the variations in the viral subtypes as well.[76] Southern and eastern Africa seem to be uniquely characterized by a very large number of migrant male workers and dislocated households, a legacy of apartheid, regional violence, and labor practices of the mining sector. These patterns most likely result in high rates of sexual contact with commercial sex workers. High levels of genital ulcer disease and low levels of male circumcision may also help to explain why the highest levels are seen in southern and eastern Africa, as opposed to west Africa. Nevertheless, no country has escaped this pandemic. HIV has spread in rich and poor countries and, within countries, among both rich and poor.

While some countries are already burdened with very high prevalence rates, others, such as China and India, are still at an early phase of the pandemic, so that timely control measures can head off an explosive growth of infections. The evidence, still incomplete, suggests a dramatic surge of HIV infections in both China and India, threatening the two most populous societies in the world. The costs of inaction in these countries could be literally tens of millions of deaths that could be averted through policies with a sense of urgency today.

The key to curbing and eventually reversing the HIV/AIDS pandemic is blocking the transmission of the virus. Regarding sexual transmission of the virus, the predominant form of transmission, there are two main strategies: reducing the number of sexual partners of people already infected, partly it is hoped through voluntary counseling and testing of those already HIV infected; and reducing the likelihood that sex between an infected and uninfected person will lead to disease, for example through the use of condoms. For transmission caused by blood exchanges, reducing the sharing of needles among injecting drug users, screening blood used for transfusions, and sterilizing injecting equipment in blood transfusions and medical procedures are all vital. For prenatal and perinatal mother-to-child transmission, the use of antiretroviral therapies has been shown to be effective. Prevention would of course be hugely helped by the development of vaccines against HIV; even vaccines of relatively low efficacy could substantially change the dynamics of the pandemic. The development of effective vaccines is thus the highest research priority in the field of HIV/AIDS. However, without a vaccine at hand there is still much that can be done to prevent the spread of the disease.

The most clearly effective preventive interventions against HIV are those that change transmission rates among groups that—because of high rates of partner change, increased susceptibility to infection, or both—are most likely to get infected and pass the virus to others. Commercial sex workers are a very important group in this regard. Around the world there have been significant successes scored through programs that seek to increase condom use among commercial sex workers, mostly through education provided by peers. First in Thailand and now in Cambodia, efforts to identify areas of commercial sex work, and then to provide peer education and treat STIs, have resulted in dramatic declines in HIV not just among the vulnerable sex workers but in the general population too. The Indian state of Tamil Nadu seems on the verge of similar success. Interventions with sex workers can be combined with improved management of other sexually transmitted infections, which can make people more vulnerable to infection. Such improved treatment seems likely to be very useful in HIV control, though divergent studies of the issue mean that more research is needed. Treatment of STIs may also provide a point of access to the clients of sex workers and other men with numerous sexual encounters. Modeling studies done for the Commission suggest that a combination of peer education programs for sex workers and their clients and STI services could hold down the eventual number of Indian AIDS deaths by tens of millions.

There is also a pressing need for programs aimed at adolescents, an especially vulnerable group. Although there is little reliable information on the efficacy of interventions with adolescents, a study in Namibia (Shanton et al. 1998) has suggested that well-designed school-based programs can help increase both the age at which adolescents first have sex and the likelihood that they will use condoms. Among adults, workplace peer education may also lead to significant behavioral change: a randomized trial of this type of intervention in Zimbabwe found a 30 percent reduction in HIV-1 incidence (Machekano 1998).

While there have been many well-documented successful pilot projects to prevent HIV, there are very few examples of successful policy affecting behavior on a national scale. When national-scale successes have been achieved, such as reducing the HIV-prevalence rate in Uganda and keeping it low in Senegal, outspoken and frank national leadership has played an important role. Many politicians, however, have run away from HIV/AIDS rather than mobilizing action against the disease. They are afraid of publicizing a fatal condition for which they lack the budgetary resources to provide solutions. Increased donor support for treatment would enable politicians to speak much more openly about prevention as well. Moreover, the transmission of the virus touches on human sexuality and the most private and intimate behaviors, as well as highly stigmatized behaviors such as injecting drug use and homosexuality. Political leaders are reluctant to engage in public discourse on these topics or to endorse highly effective policies that may be perceived by the public as supportive of socially deviant behavior (such as promotion of condom use by commercial sex workers or clean needles for injecting drug users).

A second reason for lack of success in national programs is the capacity constraints, including a shortage of human resources in government and NGOs, in the face of an enormous, complex, and diverse implementation agenda sometimes driven by donors and the international community. Trying to do too much with too few people can result in low quality and limited coverage for lots of initiatives. Additional financial resources are enormously important for scaling up capacity, including training. In the short term, selectivity and prioritization and financing of scaling up are critical if coverage, quality, and impact of those interventions are to be ensured.

At the same time that we emphasize prevention, we must provide effective treatment for the 36 million people currently living with the infection, 95 percent of whom are in developing countries. These individuals will die early and painful deaths unless they have access to appropriate medical care, which can markedly extend life. Without treatment, they will leave behind grieving families, tens of millions of orphans, and social and economic devastation in the hard-hit regions. Treatment is not just a moral necessity, but a necessary component of economic stabilization and an ultimate return to economic development in high prevalence parts of the world. It has also become much more affordable, with significant drops in prices of the necessary medications. Total annual treatment costs, including drugs and medical services, are now around $500 to $1,000 per year in sub-Saharan Africa, probably about the same as the average annual income of the prime-aged workers being struck down by the disease. This makes such treatment cost effective in the aggregate economic terms described earlier, even if still unaffordable by the individuals themselves.[77]

Treatments for some of the opportunistic infections (OIs) that contribute to HIV/AIDS mortality have been available since the mid 1980s, and some are in cost-effective use in parts of the developing world (most notably antibiotics effective against tuberculosis). Since 1996, highly active antiretroviral therapy (HAART), which acts directly on the virus, has dramatically increased the life expectancy of people receiving treatment. Note that treatment for OIs, however, will significantly extend life only in conjunction with HAART. Tragically, because of the costs of treatment, only a negligible fraction of those in low-income countries who would benefit from treatment are able to receive it. It is estimated that, of the 25 million HIV-infected Africans and the roughly 4 million each year with advanced HIV-related disease, only around 10,000 to 30,000 Africans receive antiretroviral therapy, and many of those are surely receiving an ineffective course of treatment because they can afford the drugs only sporadically. UNAIDS and WHO estimate that it will be possible to scale up coverage to around 5 million individuals in low-income settings, with substantial coverage in Africa, by the end of 2006.

Since HIV mutates readily, the widespread availability of HAART is certain to lead to an increase in drug-resistant strains of HIV. It is therefore vital that HAART interventions be managed with great care and public health methods in such a way as to minimize this development. It has been suggested that the directly observed treatment approach used in tuberculosis control might be applied to HAART, but the challenge would be qualitatively different, since HAART requires lifetime adherence. Fortunately, the complexity of the HAART regimen is being reduced significantly, for example by packaging the full combination of antiretroviral medicines into a single pill to be taken twice a day (for example, Trizivir). Because of the near inevitability of growing drug resistance, it seems that an ongoing commitment to HAART will require the introduction of new drugs over time, ideally drugs requiring ever-simpler regimens. Especially because of the concerns over drug resistance, but also more generally because HAART remains a complex regimen of a complex disease, the introduction of HAART in low-income settings should be accompanied by extensive operational research to test the effectiveness of alternative regimens and approaches. We believe that at least 5 percent, and perhaps more, of total funding for HIV/AIDS treatment should be set aside for operational research.

The introduction of treatment in low-income countries should certainly be undertaken with an eye toward bolstering prevention as well. Although treatment should be viewed primarily in medical terms (ie, prolonging lives of sick individuals) rather than in public health terms (ie, breaking the transmission of the virus), treatment programs should be designed in a way to leverage prevention efforts as well. For example, it makes sense for donor-supported programs to offer funding for treatment only in conjunction with active prevention programs, since both are necessary to combat the pandemic. Second, the availability of treatment will greatly increase the numbers of individuals coming forward for voluntary counseling and testing (VCT), once they know that treatment will be available in the event that they test positive. It is estimated that only around 5 percent of HIV-infected Africans currently know their status. That number could rise sharply in the event of increased access to treatment. With effective VCT, it may be possible to bring about behavioral change of those already infected but currently unaware of their condition. Of course, this positive outcome must be balanced against a risk that access to treatment (and a naïve belief that treatment offers a "cure") could result in more risky sexual behavior on average, including by those not yet infected. Third, it is possible, though not yet proved, that individuals on treatment (with high adherence) will themselves become less infective because of a reduced number of viruses in the body (reduced "viral load").

Both prevention and treatment are costly. Treating opportunistic infections will require substantial resources on the same order of magnitude as antiretroviral therapy. We estimate that the total costs of AIDS care could reach $14 billion by 2007 and around $22 billion by 2015, roughly divided in thirds between prevention, OI treatment, and antiretroviral therapy (see Table A2.2). This level of spending would permit around two-thirds of HIV-infected individuals in the low-income countries to be covered, as needed, by treatments for OIs and by antiretroviral therapy (see Table 7). The numbers actually under care at any point would be much less than two-thirds of the HIV-infected individuals, however, since antiretroviral therapy would apply only for patients whose immunological status (e.g., viral load and CD4 count) exceed certain clinical thresholds, and treatment for OIs would of course depend as well on the specific conditions of the patients as well. We assume that the Global Fund to Fight AIDS, Tuberculosis, and Malaria (GFATM) would pay for part, though not all, of the HIV control in low-income countries. Specifically, we have recommended that the GFATM should fund around $8 billion per year by 2007, and $12 billion per year by 2015, with the balance of needs met by other bilateral and multilateral donor programs and by domestic resources of the recipient countries.

Levels of Health Spending in Low-Income Countries

The essential interventions needed to eliminate much of the avoidable mortality of the low-income countries are not expensive, but are they not free either. A core part of the Commission's work has been to estimate the costs of scaling up critical interventions in the low-income world, defined for these purposes as all of sub-Saharan Africa plus all other countries of income less than or equal to $1,200 per person per year (see Table A2.B, for a complete list of countries and country groupings). We have also prepared the cost estimates by various sub-groupings of countries on a regional and income basis. The set of interventions, and the target levels for coverage of those interventions, are shown in Table 7. For example, it is assumed that DOTS coverage for TB treatment will rise from an estimated 44 percent of TB-infected patients to 60 percent by 2007, and then to 70 percent by 2015. These coverage numbers may look low to some; we have somewhat conservatively estimated what is feasible based on the existing levels of infrastructure and trained personnel, and assuming a bold but feasible process of health-sector investments and scaling up from this point forward. The detailed description of the set of interventions is

Table 7. COVERAGE GOALS FOR MAJOR SCALE UP (AND ESTIMATED CURRENT 2002 COVERAGE)

	2002	2007	2015
TB	44%	60%	70%
Malaria			
Treatment	31%	60%	70%
Prevention	2%	50%	70%
HIV			
Prevention (outside health sector)	10–20%	70%	80%
Prevention (within health sector)	< 1% – 10%	40%	70%
Care of OI	6%–10%	40%	70%
HAART	< 1%	45%	65%
Immunization*			
BCG/DPT/OPV	75%	90%	90%
HepB/HIB**			
Measles	68%	80%	80%
IMCI			
ARI	59%	70%	80%
Diarrhea	52%	70%	80%
Maternal			
ANC	65%	80%	90%
Skilled birth attendance	45%	80%	90%
Smoking control polices (tax greater than 80%, ad and promotion bans, consumer information)	20%	80%	80%

* includes provision of Vitamin A; ** HepB/HIB are not included in 2002 coverage.

presented in the WG5 Synthesis Report. Note that the costs aim to provide a full economic price of providing the health interventions, including the direct costs of medicines and health services, capital investments, complementary management and institutional support, and investments in training new personnel.

To reach the increased coverage rates by 2007 would require an additional $14 per person per year (2002 prices in US dollars) in the low-income countries, and $22 per person per year in the least-developed countries, on top of the existing level of expenditures in 2002. With current domestic resources of around $21 per person in the low-income countries (and just $13 per person in the least-developed countries), total expenditures by 2007 would be around $34 per person per year in the low-income countries, and $38 per person per year in 2015. We might regard this level, very roughly, as the minimum per capita sum needed to introduce the essential health interventions. It is clearly a quite modest level compared, say, with the average expenditures in the high-income countries of more than $2,000 per person per year. But it is a high level compared with current outlays, and, as we stress, it is high compared with the ability to pay of the low-income countries, especially the least-developed countries. The specific financing needs will of course vary across countries and regions, depending on the disease epidemiology (e.g., the incidence and prevalence of malaria, HIV/AIDS, and TB) and local economic conditions (reaching much higher levels in the middle income sub-Saharan African countries afflicted by HIV/AIDS). Most of the $30 to $45 will have to come through public outlays, for two reasons: to cover public goods (such as infectious disease control), where individuals lack the incentive on their own to take the necessary protective actions; and to ensure access for the poor, who lack adequate household funding.

We note that our estimate of the per capita costs of providing essential services is in line in general terms with other recent studies that have approached this issue from somewhat different perspectives. For example, David Evans, Chris Murray, and colleagues at the WHO have estimated that effective health services require around $80 per person per year in purchasing-power-parity-adjusted dollars (Evans et al. 2001). Using WHO estimates that each $1 of expenditure in a low-income country is equal to about $2 to $3 on a PPP-adjusted basis, the $80 threshold is akin to a $33 to $40 threshold in current (rather than PPP-adjusted) dollars, and thus is in line with our own estimates. Using a very different approach, cost estimates of the high-quality mission-hospital sector in Ghana also suggest that scaling up would require annual spending per covered population of around $45 per person in current dollars, not including initial capital costs for physical infrastructure (Arhin-Tenkorang and Buckle 2001). A recent study undertaken at the International Monetary Fund (IMF) suggests that effective health coverage would require around 12 percent of GNP of the low-income countries in order for the countries to meet the International Development Goals of reduced infant mortality.[78] For the least-developed countries, with annual GNP per capita of around $300 per person, this suggests spending on the order of $36 per person per year. If anything, we are on the low end of the range of estimates.

Table 8. DOMESTIC SPENDING AND DONOR ASSISTANCE ON HEALTH, 1997–1999

	Public Spending on Health (per person, 1997, $US)	Total Spending on Health (per person, 1997, $US)	Donor Assistance for Health (per person, average annual 1997–1999)	Donor Assistance for Health, annual average ($US millions 1997–1999)
Least-Developed Countries	6	11	2.29	1,473
Other Low-Income Countries	13	23	0.94	1,666
Lower-Middle-Income Developing Countries	51	93	0.61	1,300
Upper-Middle-Income Developing Countries	125	241	1.08	610
High-Income Countries	1,356	1,907	0.00	2
All Countries			0.85	5,052

Note: Unweighted averages for countries in respective categories. Includes only countries with population of 500,000 or more in 1997.

We stress, however, that not a lot of quality health services can be purchased at $30 to $45 per person, certainly not the kind of comprehensive care found in the high-income countries, where outlays are currently $2,000 or more per year![79] Our estimates refer to a rather minimal health system, one that can attend to the major communicable diseases and maternal and perinatal conditions that account for a significant proportion of the avoidable deaths in the low-income countries. Our costing estimates do not include some key categories that will need to be part of any operational health system, such as trauma and emergency care (broken bones, appendectomies); tertiary hospitals; and family planning (including distribution of contraceptives) beyond the first year after birth. We regard these estimates as an accurate though lower-end assessment of what is needed for a decisive drop in avoidable deaths due to the disease conditions on which we are focusing. Delivering these interventions effectively will, however, strengthen the capacity of local health services to respond to the daily needs of health care as well, an important precondition for poor households to increase their utilization of publicly financed health services.

Most low-income countries don't even achieve the minimally acceptable levels of services, or the spending per person needed for that. Among the 48 least-developed countries (Table 8), the unweighted average outlays for health stood at $11 per capita in 1997, of which $6 came from the budget and the rest mainly from out-of-pocket expenditures. Among the other low-income countries, average outlays were $23 per capita in 1997, still below the minimal threshold, of which around $13 came from budgetary outlays. These sums include the health outlays backed by donors. In fact, current levels of donor support are extremely low—just $2.29 per capita in the least-developed countries in 1997–1999, and $0.94 per person in the other low-income countries.

Mobilizing Greater Domestic Resources for Health

The inadequate levels of health spending are, first and foremost, a reflection of the basic arithmetic of poverty. When a country has a GNP of just $500 per person per year, even health outlays equal to 5 percent of GNP amount to merely $25 per person per year. There are 1.8 billion people living in countries with per capita income less than $500 per capita, and all but 35 million of these people live in countries that have average health outlays below $25 per person per year (the exceptions being Kenya and Nicaragua). Not a single country with income of $500 or less per year (which includes 44 countries in our data sample) managed to spend $30 per person per year on health. And not a single one of the governments in those countries raised even $20 per person per year for public outlays on health.

As shown in Figure 5, for 167 countries in 1997, health expenditures were determined mainly by national income.[80] Each 1 percent rise in income leads to a slightly more than 1 percent rise in health spending.[81] The poorest countries are shockingly poor by the standards of the high-income world, and their health spending, as a result, is shockingly low. Even if poor countries allocated more domestic resources to health, such measures would still not resolve the basic problem: poor countries lack the needed financial resources to meet the most basic health needs of their populations. At $30 to $40 per capita for essential interventions, these costs would represent more than 10 percent of GNP of the least-developed countries, far above what can in fact be mobilized out of domestic resources.

Nonetheless, the Commission examined carefully the extent to which increased domestic resources, especially budgetary resources, could be mobilized for health in low-income countries. With regard to public-sector resources, the capacity to generate increased revenues for health of course differs across countries, and is based on their economic structures, tax collection capacities, overhang of internal and external debt which

Figure 5. GRAPH OF LOG (GNP PER CAPITA, 1997) VERSUS LOG (PUBLIC HEALTH
EXPENDITURES PER CAPITA, 1997) (partial-regression plot)

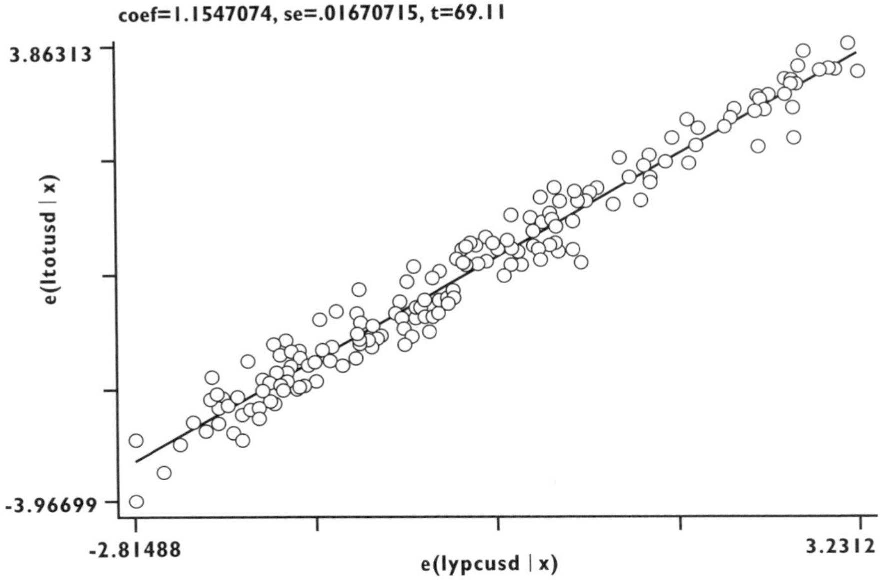

coef=1.1547074, se=.01670715, t=69.11

budgetary outlays for debt servicing, and many other factors. In general, as we see in Table 9, poorer countries mobilize a smaller share of GNP in tax revenues: an average of 14 percent of GNP in low-income countries compared with 31 percent of GNP in high-income countries. Moreover, given the limitation on raising broad-based taxes such as income tax or value-added tax, the tax collection tends to be on international trade and specific commodities, with consequent high degrees of distortion and a limited capacity to fund increases in public spending.

Still, there are cases where public spending on health is much less than could plausibly be mobilized, but the political will is not present. When societies are sharply divided, for example along geographical or ethnic lines, governments may direct public spending toward a small, favored minority rather than the broad population. Also, where there is discrimination against women, who are generally responsible for health care within the family, the result is often less attention to the health care needs of the poor in general, and of women in particular.

It's also true that the meager expenditures are frequently wasted. This is especially true of out-of-pocket spending of the poor, which goes for low-quality or inappropriate treatment. In China and India, for example,

Table 9. TAXATION AS A PERCENTAGE OF GDP

Countries	Total Tax Revenue	Taxes on International Trade	Excises	General Sales Taxes	Social Security
Low income (31) Under $760 per capita	14.0	4.5	1.6	2.7	1.1
Lower middle (36) $761–$3,030 per capita	19.4	4.2	2.3	4.8	4.0
Upper middle (27) $3,631–$9,360 per capita	22.3	3.7	2.0	5.7	5.6
High income (23) Over $9,360 per capita	30.9	0.3	3.1	6.2	8.8

Source: *Government Finance Statistics, IMF. Classification of Countries Incomes is as posted in the DAC List of Aid Recipients as of 1 January 2000. Number of countries in parentheses.*

the rural poor pay out of pocket for around 85 percent of the total health services that they receive, and much of that goes for unnecessary or inappropriate drugs foisted on them by clinics that fund themselves through sales of pharmaceutical products, or to unlicensed and unqualified practitioners.[82] High and rising health costs exclude a significant proportion of the poor from essential services, and a very large number of families are thrown into poverty each year by health outlays.[83] In Africa, many households spend enormous sums for informal and traditional forms of care with dire health consequences. Of course, some private outlays go for good treatment from the private and NGO sectors. Public outlays as well can be wasteful or misdirected, as when too much devoted funding goes toward high-tech curative services for urban elites in the capital cities, and not enough for the essential interventions to control communicable diseases for the rural poor or to respond to the basic needs for curative and maternal and child health services of the poor more generally.

Given the limited capacity of low-income countries to mobilize government revenues, and the considerable demands on those revenues for public administration, infrastructure, agriculture, police, defense, education, and debt servicing in addition to health, it is probably optimistic to expect that low-income countries could muster even 4 percent of GNP in budgetary outlays for health. In fact, that level of government outlay for health was not reached by a single country with per capita income below $600 per year.[84] Although most countries could mobilize more budgetary spending for health, it is also realistic to assume that increased revenues would not exceed more than 1 to 2 percent of GNP for the low-income countries. As an indicative guideline for our costing estimates, we have assumed that on average the low-income countries will increase their budgetary outlays on health by 1 percent of GNP as of 2007 and by 2 percent of GNP by 2015. For a country at $500 per capita, the increase would be $5 per person per year as of 2007 and $10 per person per year as of 2015, not enough to close the gap between the costs of essential services and the available resources. Some inefficiency in the health sector, both in terms of a poor allocation of resources and inefficiency in the technology used, could also be addressed, but this is likely to result in savings of no more than 20 percent of existing spending (Henscher 2001). Only donor assistance can close that financing gap for the low-income countries.

There are, in fact, two other problems with the current health-financing arrangements of the low-income countries, in addition to the insufficient overall levels of spending. First, the proportion of total health outlays coming through the budget is also relatively low (55 percent), much lower than in the high-income countries (71 percent). Since public-sector spending on health is needed to provide critical public goods (such as epidemic disease control) and to ensure enough resources for the poor to gain access to health services, the meager size of public outlays exacerbates the problem of the overall insufficiency of resources. Second, the private spending tends to be out of pocket, rather than pre-paid, so that there is very little insurance element (ie, risk pooling) built into private spending, again in contrast to the much higher rate of insurance coverage in high-income countries. Such private spending, moreover, tends to be inefficient, being spent on high-priced pharmaceuticals and poorly trained practitioners.

The Commission recommends that out-of-pocket expenditures in poor communities should increasingly be channeled into "community financing" schemes to help cover the costs of community-based health delivery. The basic idea of such arrangements is to offer local communities an incentive scheme, in which each $1 that the community raises for pre-paid health coverage would be augmented, at some rate of co-financing, by the national government (backed by donor assistance). These pre-payments by the community would mainly cover basic curative health services other than the package of essential interventions (which are to be paid for by budgetary funds, with donor support). The local community would thereby be encouraged to pool its resources, and to provide some kind of community-based oversight of health service delivery. This method would offer a degree of risk spreading, so that households would not face financial catastrophe in the event of an adverse health shock to household income. The national government would also be able to help monitor the quality of health services provided at the local level. Community-financing schemes are no panacea, and have often failed, but for many places they seem a promising and flexible mechanism that can often be harnessed to local needs.

Pre-payments in a community-financing scheme should not be confused with an alternative approach that has sometimes been tried: user fees. User fees, as conventionally defined, are payments for health services at the time of illness (that is, out-of-pocket expenditures), often levied on essential interventions. Experience has taught repeatedly that user fees end up excluding the poor from essential health services, while at the same time recovering only a tiny fraction of costs.[85] Thus the community-financing approach differs from user fees in two key respects: first, the former involves pre-payments rather than out-of-pocket expenditures, and second, contributions need not be used to cover essential services as these services would be covered by public funding that would be entirely additional to community contributions.

There is another method to raise more revenues for health in low-income countries: deeper debt relief, with the savings allocated to the health sector. The Heavily Indebted Poor Countries (HIPC) Initiative will reduce debt servicing by around 2 percent of GNP for some 30 heavily indebted poor countries, and perhaps around one-fourth of that will be allocated directly to the health sector. The debt stock will be reduced by around two-thirds in present value terms, combining traditional forms of debt reduction with the expanded relief available under the HIPC initiative. This valuable initiative could be expanded in two ways: increasing the number of countries included in the initiative, and deepening the amount of debt reduction on offer. Given the outstanding results of the first phase, in terms of channeling debt savings into social expenditure, these seem to be additional initiatives worth taking, though it would entail further bilateral financial support for a strengthening of the HIPC initiative.[86] Of course we should note that the added savings would be only a small part of the needed increment in donor assistance.

As a basic strategy for health-finance reform in the low-income countries, therefore, the Commission recommends six steps: (1) increased mobilization of general tax revenues for health, on the order of 1 percent of GNP by 2007 and 2 percent of GNP by 2015; (2) increased donor support to finance the provision of public goods and to ensure access for the poor to essential services; (3) conversion of current out-of-pocket expenditures into prepayment schemes, including community financing programs supported by public funding, where feasible; (4) a deepening of the HIPC initiative, in country coverage and in the extent of debt relief (with support from the bilateral donor community); (5) efforts to address existing inefficiencies in the way in which government resources are presently allocated and used in the health sector; and (6) reallocating public outlays more generally from unproductive expenditures and subsidies to social-sector programs focused on the poor.

The financing issues for middle-income countries are somewhat different. Total health outlays are sufficient to ensure universal access to essential health services. Two basic problems remain, however. First, many poor households within the middle-income countries nonetheless lack access to health services, since they are too poor to finance their own access and the government offers too little funding on their behalf. We strongly advise middle-income countries to mobilize the needed public finance to extend coverage to the poorest cohorts and regions. Second, the demand for coverage of interventions beyond the essential services, especially for noncommunicable diseases, puts increasing financial stress on the health system. If the payments for this growing range of services are out of pocket, then households find themselves at risk of financial ruin in the event of health shocks; and if the payments are from the budget, then rising costs of health programs become a major concern. Moreover, the mode of contracting for services (e.g., fee-for-service payments to providers versus universal access through national health insurance) makes a difference as well. Fee-for-service systems tend to lead to dramatic cost escalation, as service providers order unnecessary tests and procedures.

The experience of the high-income countries suggests that the tendency of many governments of middle-income countries to attempt to shift the finance of clinical health services to the private sector, especially via fee-for-service payments, runs the risk of dramatic cost escalation and would virtually ensure that a substantial proportion of the population will lack financial access to services in time of need. A consistent consequence of introducing universal coverage in OECD countries has been, contrary to most predictions, a leveling off in the growth rate of health expenditures as a percent of GDP during the past 10 to 15 years (Preker 1998;

Thompson and Huber 2001).[87] Preker points to the following as potential reasons: (1) greater policy control over expenditure; (2) elimination of the pressures for increased spending created by private health insurance; and (3) in some countries, close to universal coverage had been achieved prior to its introduction by legislation.

Almost all middle-income countries spend sufficient resources in the aggregate in the health sector to ensure universal access to essential services.[88] Yet this target remains unachieved in most middle-income countries because of two major reasons. First is the existence of large income inequalities within society, often along geographical or ethnic lines or both, and often coupled with a lack of political will to use public resources to ensure access for the poor. There are pockets of intense poverty in regions such as rural northeast Brazil and rural western China, and the impoverished populations there often lack access to essential interventions, with highly deleterious social and economic consequences. Second, many middle-income countries have not developed insurance for their informal sector workers. These workers pay out-of-pocket for health services and face bankruptcy when a serious illness strikes.[89] The Commission believes that as part of the economic development strategy of every middle-income country, public finances should ensure universal access to essential interventions, and this may require fiscal transfers to poorer regions earmarked for health. Public funding can also provide incentives for informal sector workers to participate in risk-pooling schemes. The experience of OECD countries in the past two decades is instructive as to how equity and efficiency can be improved through budgeting, payment, contracting, and cost containment measures.

Even if such redistributive transfers are feasible in the longer term, many middle-income countries will be strapped for cash in the short run. The World Bank and the regional development banks, working closely with the countries and with the World Health Organization, should fashion long-term loans and technical support to help these countries scale up their interventions to the poor. Even though such loans are technically nonconcessional, they offer the recipient countries better access to financing for health than would be available on the open financial markets.[90] Targeted loans from the World Bank to middle-income countries such as Brazil, China, and Thailand for AIDS and TB have demonstrated the power of this approach.

REMOVING THE NONFINANCIAL CONSTRAINTS TO HEALTH SERVICES

The constraints that deprive hundreds of millions of the world's poor of the needed access to health services go well beyond immediate funding. Most of the poorest billion people lack access to a health system that is adequate to the task. The pipes down which funds and materials might be poured are either too narrow, or clogged up, or full of holes; they may not go to the places where they are needed, or not be under the control of the health sector. There may be no pipes at all. This state of affairs—the lack of an effective and capable health delivery system—limits all efforts to scale up the provision of effective interventions. In some cases these systemic problems will become governing constraints if spending is quickly increased, driving the marginal benefit of spending on materials or staff to zero. In some parts of some developing countries this is already the case, with workers sitting idle due to dysfunctional systems.

The removal of structural constraints and the building of new capacity will typically be necessary as part of the scaling-up process. Many of these constraints can be overcome by more money, soundly used, and donors should indeed invest amply—in partnership with the recipient country—in a bold process of health system strengthening. This will take time, so it is urgent to start now to meet goals many years hence, for example by building new physical infrastructure, increasing the numbers and training of health-sector personnel, and strengthening management systems and capacity. The highest priority for scaling up is at the community level, where actual health services are delivered. We have termed this the *close-to-client*, or *CTC*, part of the health system. Scaling up at the CTC level involves a basic strengthening of the staffing at this level, an adequate supply of drugs, and a minimal capacity for transport. It also involves both the hardware of the health sector (physical plant, diagnostic equipment, telephone and e-mail connectivity of CTC centers) and the software, meaning better systems of management and supervision, and better accountability to the users through local oversight of CTC units. Without strong community involvement and trust in the CTC system, the expanded and effective coverage of the poor is unlikely to be achieved.

The state has four roles in a CTC-based delivery system. First, the state (in conjunction with institutions of civil society) would identify and justify the set of essential health interventions, based on local epidemiological conditions. Second, the state would guarantee adequate public finances (including donor support) for universal access to the set of essential interventions. Third, the state would act both as provider, in state-owned clinics and hospitals, and contractor for services, in the case of nongovernmental providers. And fourth, the state would aim to be the guarantor of quality of health service provision. In short, the state is the steward of public health, though not the sole provider in most cases. The CMH recognizes that this enhanced role of the state in the health sector would have to be realized at a time when the capacity of governments, particularly in the poorest countries, is limited, and often subject to administrative and governance constraints. Addressing these constraints will be a necessary part of the challenge faced by countries and donors alike, if the burden of ill health is to be lifted.

In organizational terms, we see the CTC system as consisting of relatively simple hospitals (not necessarily capable of the full range of interventions expected at large urban or teaching hospitals), health centers and, in some circumstances, smaller health posts. Various outreach services associated with these units will take interventions directly to the community. Though medical supervision will be necessary, a great deal of the work in this CTC part of the health system can be carried out by people other than doctors: by nurses and paramedical staff of various degrees of training, including midwives. Table 10 shows in summary form our expectation about the organizational delivery of essential services. For each intervention we indicate the presumptive organizational unit that would be the predominant provider of the service.

Hospitals within the CTC system will need to be staffed by at least one doctor and a range of paramedical staff, and may typically be capable of offering in-patient care to at least 100 people at a time. The purpose of these hospitals is to deal with acute and peculiarly dangerous or complicated cases. In the area of maternal health they would be the referral destinations for eclampsia, postpartum hemorrhaging, puerperal sepsis, and complications associated with poorly performed terminations. They would be the appropriate setting for some case management of severe cases of childhood disease and malaria, and for the treatment of complicated tuberculosis cases. Antiretroviral treatment for AIDS patients would probably best be introduced at this level. Such hospitals should have some laboratory capacity and at least one operating theater, anesthetic and X-ray facilities, and it will have an all-purpose dispensary.

A well-functioning CTC health system will require at least one and possibly two forms of facility-based access beyond the hospital setting. The principal requirement is for a set of health centers staffed primarily by nurses and trained paramedical staff. It is at the health center that most

Table 10. EXAMPLES OF INTERVENTION DELIVERY BY LEVEL OF CARE

Level of Care	TB	Malaria	HIV/AIDS	Childhood Diseases	Maternal/Perinatal	Smoking
Hospital	DOTS for complicated TB cases	Tx of complicated malaria	Blood transfusion for HIV/AIDS HAART Tx of severe OI for AIDS Palliative care	IMCI- severe cases	Emergency obstetric care	Cessation advice; pharmacological therapies for smoking
Health center/ health post	DOTS	Tx uncomplicated malaria Intermittent treatment of pregnant women for malaria	Antiretrovirals plus breast milk substitutes for prevention of mother-to-child transmission Prevention of OI, and Tx of uncomplicated OI VCT Tx of STIs	IMCI Immunization Tx of severe anemia	Skilled birth attendance Antenatal and postnatal care Family planning post partum	
Outreach services		Epidemic planning and response Indoor residual spraying	Peer education for vulnerable groups; needle exchange	Specific immunization campaigns Outreach IMCI- home management of fever		

Table 10 cont'd

Level of Care	TB	Malaria	HIV/AIDS	Childhood Diseases	Maternal/Perinatal	Smoking
(Outreach services)				Outreach micronutrients and deworming		
Outside health sector or not involving direct service delivery		Social marketing of ITNs	Condom social marketing School youth programs for HIV	Improving quality of private drug sellers School deworming and micronutrients Policies to reduce indoor air pollution, information, regulation Food fortification laws with iodine, iron, folate, potentially zinc		Higher tobacco taxes, bans on advertising and promotion and clean air laws, counter advertising

Abbreviations

OI: opportunistic infection; IMCI: integrated management of childhood illnesses; STIs: sexually transmitted infections; Tx: treatment; VCT: voluntary counseling and testing

Note: Interventions are allocated to the level that will be the predominant service provider; other levels will often also provide specific interventions (e.g., skilled birth attendance at hospital).

DOTS treatment should take place, as well as most diagnosis and treatment of uncomplicated childhood illness, plus diagnosis and referral of cases of severe disease. This is also the best site for treatment of uncomplicated malaria (though a significant amount of malaria treatment appears possible in the home, given training and appropriately packaged materials). This is also the appropriate level for the treatment of most STIs, the treatment and prophylaxis of most opportunistic infections in HIV/AIDS cases, and HIV testing with related counseling. Advice on quitting smoking and pharmacological interventions against tobacco addiction may be appropriate to this level, too. Health centers should provide appropriate settings for uncomplicated births and for the administration of nevirapine or another retroviral to reduce the risk of mother-to-child transmission of HIV. In some situations, for example where people are widely scattered, it will make sense to provide a further level, what we call the *health post*. This will provide services such as routine immunization, postpartum and antenatal care, and treatment with anti-malarials. However, where population density is high, these routine services may be provided in health centers; in more rural areas, they may be provided through peripatetic means. A CTC health system will also include a penumbra of outreach services radiating out from static facilities. These activities can include, in the case of mother and child health, antenatal visits, vaccination campaigns, micronutrient programs, presumptive treatment for worms, and training in the home management of fever and of diarrheal disease through oral rehydration. In the case of malaria, outreach can include indoor spraying and planning for coping with epidemics. Interventions also need to be delivered outside the health sector. In the area of HIV/AIDS this is required to reach vulnerable groups with peer education initiatives, which are the key to controlling the pandemic in areas of low prevalence. Social marketing approaches can be employed to increase the use of condoms and ITNs. School health programs can target particular conditions such as parasitic infections, or provide education in sexuality to reduce the risk of transmission of HIV/AIDS. The quality of treatments purchased from the retail sector can be improved though measures such as training shopkeepers and social marketing of drugs, including pre-packaging and providing easily understood treatment advice.

Historically, one way of avoiding the problems of limited capacity within health systems has been to adopt a "vertical" or categorical approach to a particular disease—such as malaria—or family of interventions—such as childhood vaccination. Such approaches have attracted a great deal of interest from many outside donors, who appreciate the centralized technical and financial control that characterizes them and their tendency to be more easily assessed. Many such programs have met with great successes both within given countries and in some cases worldwide. We would strongly advocate that categorical approaches not be dismantled; there is a great value to the concentration of expertise and commitment that drives such approaches, and we would endorse the low-income countries maintaining or establishing national programs on HIV/AIDS, malaria, TB, and perhaps other specific conditions, even as they build the CTC systems.

The need for such focused expertise to advise or complement CTC systems is evident even when the CTC systems are functioning well. It is also important, however, to see that such categorical approaches are an adjunct to the broader health service rather than an alternative to it. Moreover, given that we are advocating greatly increased coverage of a significant number of interventions, it is clearly more sensible to strengthen the health service proper to deal with these challenges than to try and build a tangle of bypasses around it. Categorical programs can provide technical assistance to the CTC level, standard disease protocols, quality-assured drugs, and monitoring and evaluation focused on specific outcomes, and they can help to build broad political support for the particular program. In many cases, infrastructures established by these categorical approaches are being used to control other high-priority diseases. Many of the industry-supported global initiatives mentioned earlier, which depend on the distribution of drugs and other commodities to large populations, have strengthened the national infrastructures needed for the CTC delivery of interventions.

Most low-income countries will need to make substantial efforts to scale up, especially in creating the CTC system and the necessary management support it will require. We examined in detail the constraints that will have to be overcome in the process,[91] classifying them (Table 11) into five categories according to the realm in which they operate: the community and household level; the health services delivery level; the health sector policy and strategic management level; overall public policy issues; and environmental characteristics. One objective is to identify the areas where the constraints are more amenable to solution through increased financing, and those where money is less the central obstacle. The areas more amenable to solution through increased financing are within the first two

Table 11. CATEGORIZATION OF CONSTRAINTS

Levels	Constraints
Community and Household Level	Lack of demand for effective interventions Barriers to use of effective interventions: physical, financial, social
Health Services Delivery Level	Shortage and distribution of appropriately qualified staff Weak technical guidance, program management and supervision Inadequate supplies of drugs and medical supplies Lack of equipment and infrastructure (including labs and communications) and poor accessibility of health services
Health Sector Policy and Strategic Management Level	Weak, overly centralized systems for planning and management Weak drug policies and supply systems Inadequate regulation of pharmaceutical and private sector and improper industry practices Lack of intersectoral action and partnership for health between government and civil society Weak incentives to use inputs efficiently and respond to user needs and preferences Reliance on donor funding that reduces flexibility and ownership; donor practices that damage country policies
Public Policies Cutting Across Sectors	Government bureaucracy Poor availability of communication and transport infrastructure

Environmental Characteristics	A. *Governance and overall policy framework*
	    Corruption, weak government, weak rule of law and enforceability of contracts
	    Political instability and insecurity
	    Low priority attached to social sectors
	    Weak structure for public accountability
	    Lack of free press
	B. *Physical environment*
	    Climatic and geographic predisposition to disease
	    Physical environment unfavorable to service delivery

Source: Hanson et al.

categories, being factors that operate at the level of the community and the system that delivers the communities' health services. Constraints in the other three levels are more centrally about governance and institutional performance, and less about money per se. Moreover, whereas lack of management capacity is a problem at all levels, some aspects can be more quickly and simply addressed at the local level, and thus are an immediate priority, whereas reforming and strengthening central government systems requires a long-term and sustained effort.

To assess the existing constraints on a country-by-country basis, we scored each low-income country according to a number of proxy indicators. Indicators of constraints included: female literacy, nurses per 100,000 citizens, existing DPT3 immunization coverage, a UNICEF measure of access to health services, World Bank measures of control of corruption and government effectiveness, and the Harvard Center for International Development's measure of the proportion of the population living in the tropics. The analysis revealed that these vary a great deal. In low-income countries, for example, the number of nurses per 100,000 varies from 5 to 874, and the proportion of people classed as having access to healthcare from 18 percent to 95 percent.

Importantly, the two low- and lower-middle-income countries, where the majority of the poorest billion live—India and China—are firmly in the least-constrained quartile. At the other end of the spectrum, the most severely constrained countries, making up the lowest quartile, include Angola, Burundi, Cambodia, Central African Republic, Chad, Democratic Republic of Congo, Eritrea, Guinea-Bissau, Haiti, Liberia, Mauritania, Niger, Nigeria, Somalia, and Yemen. Most of these countries are in sub-Saharan Africa, and many are in conflict (internally or externally) or have recently been in conflict. Many have grievous governance shortfalls. We observe a qualitative difference between these countries and those in the higher quartiles; in other countries, specific indicators of constraint are much less highly correlated with each other than they are in these most highly constrained countries.

These most-constrained countries represent the hardest cases for intervention. They have health indicators significantly worse than those for low-income countries as a whole: they have only a third of the number of nurses per capita, almost twice the infant mortality, and more than twice the maternal mortality. The proportion of their population living on less than $1 a day is twice that in other low-income countries. However, it is important to note that in absolute terms these countries represent a relatively small part of the problem. These are for the most part small countries (more than half have populations below 10 million), and their combined population is about 250 million. Despite the fact that they have high rates of poverty, they represent only 13 percent of the total population living on less than $1 a day in low-income countries. To put it another way, 87 percent of the people living on less than $1 a day in low-income countries do not live in the most highly constrained settings.

This analysis is rough, leaving out some countries in the quartile near to the bottom, where constraints weigh heavily. However, it is common in some circles to argue that nothing can be done for the poorest billion because they live in countries where governance is too poor, civil society too weak, levels of education too low, and investment in infrastructure too nugatory for outside assistance to achieve any sustainable good. This is not the case. As noted, though there are indeed places that appear too constrained for hope in this way, most of the poor do not live in such places, but in countries where the situation is appreciably better. Substantial investments in capacity building in order to address constraints will still be required even in countries well above the lowest quartile in order for additional funding to be used effectively.

There is an argument to be made, in fact, that a poor climate for development in general—poor governance, a weak economy, rampant corruption, and so on—is a bit less of a hindrance to targeted health programs than to some other forms of development assistance. Smallpox eradication required effective interventions in all countries regardless of constraints; more recently the Onchocerciasis Control Programme (OCP) has achieved significant goals in highly constrained settings, as has been the case with leprosy, guinea-worm disease, Chagas disease, and other initiatives backed by robust interventions. The lesson in these cases is important: international programs—supplied as global public goods—were needed to overcome domestic barriers. Provision of health interventions at the international scale may sometimes substitute for weak domestic political systems.

Another consideration is that conditions of high constraint are occasionally transitory. Had our analysis been carried out a few years earlier, countries such as Uganda and Mozambique would probably have been found among the most constrained. Today they have considerable successes to of which to boast. What we are identifying as highly constrained countries are in many circumstances what others would refer to as complex emergencies, where the high constraints are due to exceptional circumstances. Complex emergencies are not permissive environments for health interventions, but they are environments that require them, especially in terms of epidemic control, for malaria and for other diseases. In those cases where the underlying governance situation improves, money spent on categorical health programs in such situations may yield institutional capacity useful for more generalized improvements in the health system.

Still, national governance that is marked by corruption, a lack of planning, and a lack of concern for long-term development will undermine the health sector as well as the rest of the economy. Countries in violent conflict, or that repress ethnic or racial minorities, or that discriminate against girls and women, will find it difficult or impossible to make sustained improvements in health sector capacity. Countries that centralize power in authoritarian institutions and deprive local communities of power and participation in their own affairs, including health, will also fall far short of the potential gains. We cannot easily quantify the proportion of countries that fall into these cases: they exist, and not in small number, alas. It would do no good to the overall effort of scaling up health interventions if the donors put large sums into such countries, only to see the efforts wasted and the donor taxpayers lose confidence.

Short-term macroeconomic crises can gravely damage access to health services and upset the process of scaling up those services, unless the sector is well insulated from short-term shocks. Donor agencies and multilateral institutions, in concert with country officials, need to give special attention to protecting essential health interventions from budgetary austerity that might accompany a short-run macroeconomic crisis. Donor support can be a critical tool in that task of sustaining essential health services during economic downturns. Preemptive efforts to formulate social safety net schemes are equally critical to protect the poor in such situations; if households are thrown into poverty, simply maintaining the level of essential health services that existed before the economic downturn cannot prevent adverse health effects.

PLACING THE HEALTH SECTOR INTO A BROADER CONTEXT OF HEALTH PROMOTION

An effective health policy requires a detailed understanding of local conditions—ecological, social, demographic, economic, and political—that all affect health, and that need to be addressed in a public health strategy. Important investments and behavioral changes are needed in many key areas beyond the health sector itself (as least as traditionally defined). Econometric estimates of health outcomes prepared for this Report (specifically, female life expectancy in a panel of countries, 1975 to 1990) confirm the multiple roles of health and medical services (as measured by number of doctors per capita), household income (proxied by per capita GNP), and ecological conditions (tropical locations adverse for health, coastal locations favorable for health).[92] Beyond the reform of the health sector, health policy should address at least four areas.

(1) Underlying Infrastructure and Technology for Health

Even before the advent of some of the most potent health interventions of the 20th century, such as immunizations and antibiotics, life expectancy began to rise and morbidity to decline in western Europe and North America. These gains were achieved through improvements in what Fogel has termed the "health infrastructure," including improved access to clean water; urban sewage and garbage disposal services; pasteurized milk and other safety precautions in food preparation and storage, and increased nutrient intake, especially following improvements in agricultural technology and productivity; and reduced transport costs of bringing food to urban centers. We stress that improved infrastructure is not merely the bricks and mortar, but the know-how as well. Critical investments are needed in technological advancement not only in biomedical approaches but also in agriculture (e.g., nutritionally fortified crops, or higher-yielding crops), environmental management, and other areas.

(2) Ecological Conditions

Many diseases are heavily conditioned by the physical ecology of a country. Diseases depend on temperature, rainfall, availability of clean water supplies, the presence of specific disease vectors such as mosquitoes (which in turn are affected by climate, accident of history, biogeography), the density of habitation (or the crowding of individuals), exposure to environmental risks such as indoor air pollution or unsafe water, and so forth. Islands are different from mainlands,[93] temperate zones are different from tropical zones, humid regions are different from deserts, coasts are different from hinterlands. It is not surprising that malaria has been defeated in most temperate regions but not in large parts of the tropics; or that Africa suffers the most intensive malaria transmission, in part because it also has the most pernicious (or "competent") mosquito vector (*Anopheles gambiae*). Hot environments and seasons are much more prone to bacterial-induced diarrheal diseases than cooler regions and seasons. Costs and strategies may differ markedly according to ecology, and intervention strategies must be tailored to local ecological conditions.[94] In some regions, insecticide-impregnated bednets might be the best vector-control response to malaria; in other places, household spraying or larviciding of breeding sites might be more effective.

(3) Social Conditions, Including Education and Gender Equality

Social conditions matter enormously. Literacy, for example, particularly female literacy, contributes importantly to good health. Some societies ensure widespread literacy. Others deny literacy to girls, and still others deny literacy to ethnic minorities or low-status social groups. Thus, ethnic divisions, social stratification, and gender discrimination may play a large role in the success or failure of disease control. Women's social status is a major determinant of health outcomes. Women have been shown in many societies to invest the household's scarce economic resources in their children's health and education than do men. The mother's literacy is critical for almost any health interventions, whether personal behaviors or access to the formal health care system. Once again, societies that limit girls' access to education pay a price in poorer health, and thereby in poorer economic growth. Thus it is important to ensure that poor women and girls have equitable access to information, services, and medicines. They should also play an important role in the involvement of the community and civil society that we recommend here. In sum, the MDG calling for gender equality and empowerment of women—which includes but is not limited to equality in education—is important for achieving the MDGs on health, and for the initiative recommended here.

Sexual practices may strongly influence the patterns of spread of sexually transmitted disease. We have noted that the high prevalence of AIDS in Africa is a result, in part, of sexual networks with significant groups of high-risk individuals, such as male migrant workers (e.g., miners) who frequent commercial sex workers. Furthermore, women's lack of power in sexual relations in Africa and parts of Asia may amplify the transmission of the HIV virus. Another culturally determined factor, male circumcision (especially prevalent in Muslim societies in Africa), may be protective against HIV transmission, as evidenced by the lower prevalence rates in predominantly Muslim countries in west Africa.

(4) Globalization

Globalization overall offers potential health benefits to all of the world (Feachem 2001). A more integrated global market is likely to increase the rate of innovation and diffusion of technological advance (for example, through trade in health services), and this could surely serve for the common benefit of humanity. Still, the low-income countries face at least four policy challenges arising from globalization. First, globalization has probably intensified the problem of brain drain from the poorest countries. It is estimated that in the case of 20 African countries—Algeria, Benin, Burkina Faso, Cape Verde, Côte d'Ivoire, Gambia, Ghana, Guinea, Guinea Bissau, Liberia, Mali, Mauritania, Morocco, Nigeria, Senegal, Sierra Leone, Somalia, Sudan, Togo, and Tunisia—more than 35 percent of nationals with a university education are now living abroad (International Organization for Migration 2001). As Africa struggles with the out-migration of doctors, high-income countries such as Canada and the United States actively recruit these doctors with special inducements, visa preferences, and advertising campaigns. Second, with increased competition for internationally mobile capital, many governments are finding that they must lower tax rates to compete internationally for investment. These tax cuts may, on balance, be beneficial for economic growth, but they make it harder for governments to finance public expenditures for health. Some countries, such as China, took decisions that required local health centers to cover an increasing fraction of their budgets out of market revenues, thus excluding the poor from access to essential services (and inducing these centers to oversupply drugs and other services by which they could cover their costs). Third, globalization is most likely increasing the pace of international transmission of diseases. Theoretical studies suggest that even modest increases in international linkages across populations (e.g., due to tourism, migration, or business travel) could substantially increase the rate of transmission of infectious diseases.[95] Fourth, globalization is undercutting many local cultural patterns, related for example to diet and drug use. We are witnessing rapid increases in unhealthy practices such as high-fat-content foods, increased tobacco use, and increased use of illicit drugs (which may also be major channels for transmitting AIDS, hepatitis C, and other blood-borne diseases).

THE SUPPLY OF GLOBAL KNOWLEDGE IN THE FIGHT AGAINST DISEASE
Public goods, in the broadest terms, are kinds of economic activities and products that are undersupplied by the market, and therefore require public provision and/or financing. When public goods are local (such as police and fire protection) or national (such as public defense), local or national governments, respectively, are the key providers. Global Public Goods (GPGs) are public goods that are underprovided by local and national governments, since the benefits accrue beyond a country's borders. The fight against disease requires important investments in GPGs, beyond the means or incentives of any single government and beyond the sum total of national-level programs.

One of the most important kinds of public goods are those that involve the production of new knowledge, especially through investments in research and development (R&D). Since knowledge is "non-rival," meaning that the use of knowledge by one person does not diminish its availability for others, it makes sense for society to ensure that new knowledge is widely available and actually used. Yet if the fruits of R&D are freely available, profit-maximizing firms will lack the incentive to invest in R&D in the first place. The pragmatic approach in balancing the need for availability of knowledge with the need for private incentives to invest in R&D is to combine two policy instruments: public financing of R&D in combination with patent protection for private investors in R&D. In the United States, for example, the federally funded biomedical research supported by the National Institutes of Health (NIH) plays a vital role in new drug development, feeding into the R&D activities of the private pharmaceutical industry that operates under patent protection.

The division of labor in R&D between the public and private sectors is related, at least in principle, to the nature of the knowledge that is fostered. Specifically, it is not advisable for society to grant patent rights to basic scientific knowledge, since society benefits from the widespread use and dissemination of basic scientific ideas.[96] Thus, public support for R&D for basic scientific research is absolutely essential. Even in the "free market" United States, there is strong bipartisan support for this kind of public spending.[97] On the other hand, for specific applications of broad scientific concepts, patent protection gives the incentive for product development and testing, which is both risky and expensive. Since patents are given on applications rather than basic knowledge, competition among patent holders is preserved by multiple and competing applications of the same freely available knowledge. Viewing technological innovation as a process going from basic science to final-product testing, public financing should cover much of the initial stages while patent protection should provide incentives for the later stages of the process. When we turn to R&D directed at diseases specific to the poor countries, the incentive mechanisms fail at both ends. Poor-country governments lack the means to subsidize R&D, and patent protection means little when there is no significant market at the end of the process. The result is that the R&D for diseases specific to poor countries—such as malaria or other tropical parasitic diseases—tends to be grossly underfinanced. The poor countries benefit from R&D mainly when the rich also suffer from the same diseases![98]

It is helpful to distinguish between three types of diseases. *Type I diseases* are incident in both rich and poor countries, with large numbers of vulnerable population in each. Examples of communicable diseases include measles, hepatitis B, and *Haemophilus influenzae* type b (Hib), and examples of noncommunicable diseases abound (e.g., diabetes, cardiovascular diseases, and tobacco-related illnesses). In the case of Type I diseases, the incentives for R&D exist in the rich country markets (both through public financing of basic science and patent protection for product development). Products get developed, and the main policy issue, vis-à-vis the poor countries, is access to those technologies, which tend to be high priced and under patent protection. Many vaccines for Type I diseases have been developed in the past 20 years but have not been widely introduced into the poor countries because of cost. *Type II diseases* are incident in both rich and poor countries, but with a substantial proportion of the cases in the poor countries. R&D incentives exist in the rich country markets, therefore, but the level of R&D spending on a global basis is not commensurate with disease burden. HIV/AIDS and tuberculosis are examples: both diseases are present in both rich and poor countries, but more than 90 percent of cases are in the poor countries. In the case of vaccines for HIV/AIDS, substantial R&D is underway as a result of rich-country market demand, but not in proportion to global need or addressed to the specific disease conditions of the poor countries. In the case of TB the situation is even worse, with very little R&D underway for new and better treatment. *Type III diseases* are those that are overwhelmingly or exclusively incident in the developing countries, such as African sleeping sickness (trypanosomiasis) and African river blindness (onchocerciasis). Such diseases receive extremely little R&D, and essentially no commercially based R&D in the rich countries. When new technologies are developed, they are usually serendipitous, as when a veterinary medicine developed by Merck (ivermectin) proved to be effective in control of onchocerciasis in humans.

Some diseases straddle two categories, particularly if treatment and/or prevention is sensitive to distinct strains in rich and poor countries. AIDS falls between Type I and Type II, and malaria falls between Type II and Type III.[99] Still, the basic principle that R&D tends to decline relative to disease burden in moving from Type I to Type III diseases is a robust empirical finding. Type II diseases are often termed *neglected diseases* and Type III diseases *very neglected diseases*.

One gauge of R&D neglect is the share of total spending on a disease relative to the global burden of disease (measured, for example, as R&D spending per DALY[100]). Consider the case of malaria. Malaria accounts for around 3 percent of the total global burden of disease, as measured by disability-adjusted life years (45 million DALYs out of a world total of 1.4 billion DALYs), with more than 99 percent of the burden in the developing world. Total biomedical research of the public and private sectors is estimated to be around $60 billion per year, or $42 per DALY. Malaria research outlays are perhaps $100 million, or $2.2 per DALY.[101] Thus, the malaria R&D per DALY is around one-twentieth of the global average. It is notable and disturbing that the premier public-private partnership for developing new malaria drugs, the Malaria Medicines Venture (MMV), currently disburses less than $10 million per year in funding, and is so limited in funding that it currently aims for only $30 million per year by 2004. The WHO, in cooperation with the international pharmaceutical industry, has recently determined that for several important diseases of the poor, there is currently very little private industry R&D effort despite the scientific promise of breakthroughs in new drugs, vaccines, and diagnostics. Such neglected areas include malaria, tuberculosis, lymphatic filariasis, onchocerciasis, leishmaniasis, schistosomiasis, African trypanosomiasis and Chagas disease.[102]

The imbalance of research between diseases of the poor (Type II and especially Type III diseases) and of the rich has been recognized and documented for more than a decade. A widely read report in 1990 of the Commission on Health Research and Development noted what became known as the *90/10 disequilibrium*: that only 10 percent of R&D spending is directed at the health problems of 90 percent of the world's population. It is interesting that the original report actually put the imbalance at 95/5, which is probably more realistic.[103] This report led to the creation in 1996 of the Global Forum for Health Research, which continues to document the profound insufficiency of research effort on diseases of the poor. Many initiatives have been launched or continued to address the imbalance, but they remain profoundly underfunded. The flagship Tropical Disease Research (TDR) program of the WHO, UNDP, and World Bank, despite its many significant accomplishments in tropical disease control, is budgeted at only around $30 million per year to cover a program that includes eight major tropical diseases.[104] The Initiative for Vaccine Research (IVR), a program that pulls together all of vaccine R&D capabilities of both WHO and UNAIDS, has only around $8 million

Table 12. PRIORITIES FOR RESEARCH AND DEVELOPMENT FOR NEW DRUGS FOR POOR-COUNTRY DISEASES

Disease	Mortality per Year	Limitations of Existing Drugs	New Drugs Needed; Scientific feasiblity	Industry Currently Engaged in R&D
Malaria	1–2 million	Acquired drug resistance of existing treatments, and high costs of new treatments	Yes; High feasibility	Low, other than in MMV (public-private partnership)
TB	2 million	Acquired drug resistance, difficult compliance (duration and complexity)	Yes; High feasibility, but with long development time	Low
Lymphatic filariasis and onchocerciasis	Few deaths, but medium to high social costs	Drugs do not kill all stages of parasite; rapid reinfection	Yes; High feasibility	Low
Leishmaniasis	57,000	Acquired drug resistance, poor compliance	Yes; High feasibility	Low (except in partnership with TDR)
Schistosomiasis	14,000	Acquired drug resistance	Yes; WHO optimistic about feasibility, industry less	None
African trypanosomiasis	66,000	Acquired drug resistance, not active against all stages of the disease	Yes; WHO optimistic about feasibility, industry less	None
Chagas Disease	21,000	Not active against all stages of the disease	Yes; High feasibility for chronic infection	Low to None

Note: This table focuses on drug development rather than vaccine development, and excludes conditions such as Shigellosis, Japanese encephalitis, and dengue, where vaccines as opposed to drugs are likely to be most effective.

Source: WHO-IFPMA Roundtable (Table 11, "Priorities Infection Diseases for which additional R&D is required").

annually at its disposal to accelerate the development and availability of vaccines against no less than 13 diseases plus generic technologies to improve immunization.[105] A similar multi-agency effort in reproductive health, entitled the Special Programme of Research, Development and Research Training in Human Reproduction (HRP) has been budgeted at around $20 million per year (or $40 million per biennium). More recently, several public-private partnerships have been created, often under the initiative of the Gates and Rockefeller Foundations, to address R&D for malaria, AIDS, and TB. The level of funding for these initiatives is still very modest, despite being a great advance over earlier years.

The World Health Organization and the Global Forum for Health Research should work together with the donor and research communities to identify, on an ongoing basis, the high-priority areas of R&D for poor-country disease conditions that are neglected by the international pharmaceutical sector. Areas recently identified as priorities include vaccines for malaria, TB, and AIDS; microbicides for AIDS; new pesticides to control vector-borne diseases; and combination therapies for malaria needed to slow the onset of drug resistance to anti-malaria medicines.[106] Very neglected diseases include lymphatic filariasis, leishmaniasis, schistosomiasis, trypanosomiasis, and Chagas disease. A detailed evaluation of R&D priorities and feasibility for new drugs, undertaken by the WHO – IFPMA Roundtable, is summarized in Table 12. One of the consistent problems with these and other tropical infectious diseases is that, even when effective treatments have existed in the past, the spread of drug resistance is rendering the standard approaches ineffective, with few or no back-up (or low-cost) treatments available. The need to develop improved drugs and replacement drugs is therefore continuous. For some bacterial diseases, such as dysentery, drug resistance has become a major impediment to treatment. Note that Table 12 lacks mention of conditions where vaccines, rather than drugs, are likely to be necessary, such as shigellosis, Japanese encephalitis, and dengue, all of which are targeted by the WHO/UNAIDS Initiative for Vaccine Research.

We believe that at least $3.0 billion per year should be allocated toward R&D directed at the health priorities of the world's poor. Of that amount, $1.5 billion per year should be allocated toward targeted R&D for new drugs, vaccines, diagnostics, and intervention strategies against HIV/AIDS, malaria, TB, reproductive health, and other priority health conditions of the poor. With regard to AIDS, for example, this would include research on the use of antiretrovirals in low-income settings, vaccines for the specific viral subtypes that are prevalent in the low-income countries, and microbicides to block the transmission of the virus. Sustained flows of R&D support will be absolutely vital, since break-throughs in these areas will require years of substantial investigation and clinical trials. Both the WHO and the Global Forum for Health Research have an important role to play in overseeing the effective allocation of these increased funds.

In addition to targeted R&D, there is a need for greatly increased basic scientific research in health (e.g., epidemiology, health economics, health systems, and health policy) and biomedical topics (e.g., virology) vis-à-vis the poor countries. The Commission proposes a $1.5 billion annual expenditure for a new Global Health Research Fund (GHRF). The GHRF would act in health and biomedical research akin to the Consultative Group for International Agricultural Research (CGIAR) in the area of agriculture. The GHRF would support peer-reviewed scientif-ic research through a newly created international version of the National Institutes of Health (NIH) in the United States and/or the Medical Research Councils (MRC) of other countries. The NIH and the MRCs of the OECD countries, and MRCs in countries such as Brazil, Malaysia, and South Africa, have substantial accumulated experience in the funding of good research and in maintaining quality, transparency, and accountabili-ty. This wealth of experience must be fully tapped in the design and cre-ation of the new international NIH/MRC. Lessons from TDR, IVR, and HRP must also be considered, and it may be desirable, eventually, to sub-sume these entities within the new structure. The existing Global Forum for Health Research could play a useful role in the establishment and per-haps eventual operation of the Global Health Research Fund (GHRF).

A key goal of the GHRF would be to build long-term research capac-ity in developing countries themselves. The GHRF would provide vital funding for research groups in low-income countries. Still, a consequential buildup of research capacity must start with governments in low-income countries recognizing the importance of strengthening universities and other research-based institutions. Beyond the funding from the GHRF, new thinking is required to overcome the ubiquitous problems of low salary, institutional weakness, lack of peer review, and the brain-drain of the brightest and the best to Europe and North America. Finally, the WHO should work together with the global research-based pharmaceuti-cal industry to operationalize technology transfer to poor countries. All major research pharmaceutical companies should be encouraged to establish long-term research and training partnerships in the developing world, following for example the recent commitment of Pfizer to establish an Academic Alliance for AIDS Care and Prevention at Makarere University in Uganda, which will train African doctors on the use of AIDS medicines.

In addition to these outlays, funding will be needed for operational research as treatment efforts are scaled up in the low-income countries. Operational research involves the investigation of health interventions in practice, including issues of patient acceptability of treatment regimens and adherence to those regimens, toxicity, dosing, and modes and costs of delivery. The goal is to optimize the treatment regimen to local conditions, and to identify how best to integrate the regimen into existing services. The issue of operational research is typically neglected in country programs. The Commission urges bilateral agencies, the World Bank, and the new Global Fund to Fight AIDS, Tuberculosis, and Malaria to ensure that an adequate proportion of their country-specific project assistance is devoted to developing research capacity and conducting operational research on relevant topics. We suggest that a minimum of 5 percent of project assistance should be devoted to research relevant to the project. For example, the new Global Fund to Fight AIDS, Tuberculosis, and Malaria should vigorously support in-country research on the evaluation and improvement of the interventions against AIDS, TB, and malaria that it will be funding. A second example concerns the World Bank. Most World Bank concessional loans contain line items for operational research relevant to the project being funded or to the preparation of a subsequent project. Typically, these monies are either poorly spent, underspent, or both. The Commission calls for the Bank to ensure the effective use of these research resources, so that the necessary operational research is conducted and that local research capacity is supported and strengthened.

The Commission also supports recent discussions in the United States and Europe to modify existing orphan drug laws to stimulate R&D activity in priority areas. Orphan drug laws traditionally provide incentives to stimulate private sector R&D activity for the "rare"[107] diseases that affect a small number of people, and for which sales are not likely to turn a profit without additional incentives. These laws have been remarkably successful at attracting private-sector involvement to areas that had been previously ignored, and there is good evidence to suggest that similar mechanisms may work for diseases of the poor. Modification of existing drug laws should place special emphasis on diseases that are exclusively concentrated in the poor tropical countries, by adjusting the particular package of incentives for that purpose through tax credits, research grants, and extended patent protection.

Just as the rich countries rely both on the combination of R&D subsidies and market forces (albeit based on patents) to deliver new knowledge all the way from basic science to product development, so too the increased subsidization of R&D should be combined with market forces to help ensure that scientific breakthroughs find their way out of the laboratory and in to the clinics. The closest analogy to patent protection would be a mechanism to ensure a producer of a new product that a sufficient market exists to earn a return on product development (including the clinical trials). Although no simple institutional mechanism can be designed for this purpose, the Commission looks favorably upon innovative proposals by which the donor world would make precommitments to purchase new effective treatments and vaccines at a price that would merit the investments in product development. As an example, the new Global Alliance for Vaccines and Immunizations, which is funding vaccine purchases, could precommit to spend $10 per dose for an effective malaria, TB, or AIDS vaccine.[108] That precommitment, in combination with substantial donor funding of R&D, could persuade the pharmaceutical industry to invest much more heavily in new product development. Similarly, the Global Fund to Fight AIDS, Tuberculosis, and Malaria could announce precommitments to purchase new drugs against AIDS, malaria, and TB at sufficient prices to stimulate private-sector product development. Another mechanism would be the existing orphan drug laws in the rich countries, which give added financial incentives (e.g., tax breaks or favorable intellectual property rights provisions) to R&D on diseases with low incidence, such as unusual genetic disorders; this legislation could be extended to provide similar incentives for diseases of high incidence in poor countries and low incidence in the rich countries.

We need to harness the new information technologies to this cause as well. The internet now makes it possible to distribute medical and scientific journal articles and other information in a low-cost, rapid manner to all places with basic hardware and connectivity. Provision of such equipment should be an important element of any donor-supported plan for improving health care based on modern information. The possibilities opened up by the internet can overcome a traditional deficiency of medical research—the difficulty of delivering information to individuals in poor countries and those not associated with affluent institutions. Although many journals now put their content in an electronic form, only recently have some begun to release their articles to be used freely (gener-ally after a 6-month to 2-year delay after publication) and to provide their articles for free in the poorest countries. The recent announcement of such actions, coordinated by the WHO and the UN, by six major publishers is very welcome, but it falls far short of meeting enormous needs in many countries of slightly or appreciably greater affluence, and many important journals are not included in this initiative. For the longer run, the Commission recommends some important and feasible goals: develop-ment of large electronic archives, where millions of articles can be stored, accessed, and fully searched with many key words; a shift in the business plan for most journals, so that costs are borne by advanced countries and distribution is free, instantaneous, and worldwide via the internet; and an agreement by all journals to release their content for free distribution, archiving, and text searching within 6 months after publication, even if they continue with traditional publishing practices.

Adding up the R&D components, the Commission therefore calls for increasing R&D in six major ways: (1) $1.5 billion in annual funding through a new Global Health Research Fund (GHRF) for basic biomed-ical and health research; (2) $1.5 billion in annual funding for existing institutions that aim at new vaccine and drug development, such as TDR, IVR, and HRP (all at WHO), and the public-private partnerships for HIV/AIDS, malaria, and TB, and other diseases of the poor; (3) increased outlays for operational research at the country level in conjunction with the scaling up of essential interventions, equal to at least 5 percent of country program funding; (4) expanded availability of free scientific information on the internet, with donor-supported efforts to increase the physical connectivity of universities and other research sites in the low-income countries; (5) modification of the orphan drug legislation in the high-income countries to include the diseases of the poor; and (6) pre-commitments to purchase targeted technologies (such as vaccines for HIV/AIDS, malaria, and TB) as a market-based incentive, especially for later-stage product development.

In addition to R&D, there are other kinds of health public goods activities that require public subsidies, such as standard setting for public health, disease surveillance, and the promotion of best practices in health interventions. In the rich countries, such activities are carried out by pub-lic institutions, such as the Food and Drug Administration and the Centers for Disease Control in the United States. In the poor countries, such activ-ities tend to be dismally underfinanced if carried out at all. And with respect to health issues that cross national borders, the World Health Organization plays a unique role in international standard setting,[109] data gathering and analysis, disease surveillance, and the promotion of best practices in public health through the dissemination of best international practices. Yet in these areas, as in R&D on diseases of the poor, the level of international funding is insufficient to the global challenge.

It is not easy to get a comprehensive picture of current spending on global public goods through the WHO and other agencies. The WHO budget averaged $864 million per year during 1997 to 1999, divided almost evenly between the core budget and extra-budgetary funds. Other international agencies (UNICEF, UNFPA, UNDP, World Bank) also provide global public goods for health in addition to country-level projects, though the precise division between GPGs and national-level programs is not easily determined. In view of the urgency of scaling up global public goods in several areas—disease surveillance, epidemiological baselines, analysis and dissemination of best practices, and training at the global level—we suggest a phased increase in spending on these non-R&D global public goods on the order of an extra $1 billion per year by 2007 and an extra $2 billion by 2015, in support of the role of these and other such agencies in the initiative proposed here.

ACCESS TO ESSENTIAL MEDICINES

The poor lack access to essential medicines for many reasons, all of which must be addressed in a comprehensive manner. The most important reason, by far, is poverty itself, which means that neither the poor nor their governments can afford to purchase the essential medicines, or ensure their proper use in well-run health systems. In addition, poor people may be unaware of life-saving options because community outreach by the health service is inadequate. Access is hindered by a severe shortage of doctors and other health workers trained to select, prescribe, and use the available medicines in an efficacious manner. Some obstacles are self-imposed. Many low-income countries impose import duties and domestic taxes on essential medicines. Governments may also hinder access through burdensome procurement systems and regulatory procedures that unduly delay the use of the needed medicines.[110]

All of this is true even of drugs not covered by patents as well as patent-protected drugs. For example, many antiretroviral drugs for HIV/AIDS are not covered by patents in sub-Saharan Africa.[111] Many of the antiretroviral drugs are now available at low prices, either from generics producers or from US and European pharmaceutical patent-holders that are offering the drugs on a no-profit basis. Some drugs have even been offered for free, such as Boehringer Ingelheim's offer of nevirapine to reduce mother-to-child-transmission of HIV/AIDS. Nonetheless, in the absence of large-scale donor support, poor countries in sub-Saharan Africa with high HIV/AIDS prevalence have been unable to avail themselves, at any significant scale, of these lower prices. The same problems are observed in the access to TB drugs, even those that are off patent, as well as many vaccines that are off patent yet still too expensive for use in the low-income countries in the absence of adequate donor financing.

When adequate donor financing is available, drug pricing by pharmaceutical companies (especially for drugs under patent) can be a significant obstacle.[112] At least some essential medicines are under patent, and others that are off patent are still supplied by only a few producers. In such circumstances, producers tend to maintain high profit margins (prices far above production cost), especially in their rich-country markets. Such profit margins are the basic mechanism by which R&D outlays are recouped, and so should be recognized as part of the normal innovation process. Yet access to drugs in poor countries requires prices at or close to production cost, since the poor (and donors on their behalf) cannot afford patent-protected prices.[113] The likelihood that essential medicines will be covered by patents will increase after 2005, when all member countries of the World Trade Organization are required to put into force a harmonized patent system that includes pharmaceutical products.[114] Moreover, in the event of a substantial increase in donor funding for low-income countries, firms that might previously have decided against taking out a patent for their products may decide to do so on new drugs as a negotiating tactic vis-à-vis the donors. At the same time, we should recognize that the extension of intellectual property rights is likely to strengthen the research-based pharmaceutical industries in Brazil, China, India, and South Africa, which can certainly be a net plus if that increased R&D effort within the developing world is combined with special attention to the needs of the poor.

In principle, the patent-holding producers should be willing to price discriminate between the high-income and low-income markets to enable consumers in both markets to be served. In practice, however, the pharmaceutical companies are often reluctant to cut their prices in the low-income countries for several reasons: (1) fear that differential prices will undermine their prices in the high-income markets (either through the re-export of cheap drugs or a backlash of consumers and politicians in the high-income countries); (2) recognition by the companies that little or nothing is to be gained in terms of profits by providing drugs at cost in low-income countries; and (3) the fact that profits can actually be higher in some low-income markets as the result of a few high-priced sales to a narrow segment of rich customers as opposed to broad-based sales at close-to-production cost.

The best solution will be for the global community to establish differential pricing in low-income markets as the operational norm, not the exception.[115] The pharmaceutical industry seems increasingly prepared for such an approach, if there are sufficient assurances that low prices in low-income markets will not undermine market pricing and patent protection in the high-income markets. Several major pharmaceutical companies holding patents on antiretrovirals for HIV/AIDS have agreed to provide their products on a no-profit basis. In a recent case, a major producer announced its intention to license voluntarily its antiretroviral drugs.[116] Several major companies responded institutionally to calls by UNAIDS and WHO for improved access to antiretrovirals in a program launched in May 2000 called the Accelerated Access Initiative.[117] The companies were also spurred by AIDS activists, high-visibility competition from generics producers, and threats by Brazil and other middle-income countries to invoke compulsory licensing to produce antiretrovirals under patent.[118] International efforts, led by WHO and its partners, have secured price cuts in some cases of over 90 percent for the supply of drugs to treat multidrug-resistant TB. In a new wave of public-private partnerships, these examples are augmented by many impressive cases of drug donations to poor countries by major pharmaceutical companies for disease control efforts including African trypanosomiasis, onchocerciasis, and malaria, and for the global elimination of leprosy, lymphatic filariasis, and blinding trachoma.[119] Time-limited elimination drives have proved especially effective in recent years in attracting donations.

The pharmaceutical industry and the international community should now agree to a more general framework for action. The companies rightly insist that drug pricing is not the only obstacle to drug access. A complete international framework should therefore address the broad range of problems, including donor funding for purchase and proper utilization of the drugs, drug pricing by the pharmaceutical industry, recipient country commitments to an appropriate regulatory regime for the utilization of drugs, safeguards against counterfeiting and black-market re-exports of discounted or donated drugs, and agreements by governments of high-income countries not to push their own demands for drug discounts in the high-income markets on price discounts offered to low-income countries.

In our view, the best next step forward would be for WHO, the pharmaceutical industry (both patent holders and generic producers), and the low-income countries to agree jointly to guidelines for pricing and licensing of production in low-income markets. The guidelines would provide for transparent mechanisms of differential pricing that would target low-income countries. The guidelines would identify, a designated set of essential medicines (e.g., for AIDS, malaria, TB, respiratory and diarrheal diseases, and vaccine-preventable diseases) to low-income countries at the "lowest viable commercial prices."[120] The industry would agree to license their technologies to producers of high-quality generics for use within low-income countries whenever they choose not to supply those markets themselves or whenever the generics producers can demonstrate that they can produce the drugs at high quality and at a markedly lower cost (low enough, relative to the patent holders, to cover the costs of a modest royalty payment to the patent-holding company). The low-income countries would undertake their own reciprocal obligations, including: (1) prevention of re-export of low-priced drugs, either legally or via the black market, to high-income countries; (2) removal of other obstacles to market access, such as tariffs and quotas on the importation of essential medicines; (3) regulation and cooperation with the donor community to ensure the effective use of the medicines in order to limit the onset of drug resistance or other adverse outcomes that can accompany poor administration of medicines. The donor community, on its side, would guarantee adequate financing for the purchase, monitoring, and safe use of the drugs.

One specific mechanism would be a system of "best price wins" in international tenders by donors on behalf of low-income countries. This system calls for bidding among competing suppliers, including the patent holder and pre-approved generics producers (with approval based on the demonstrated ability to deliver high-quality products on the required scale and timetable). In case the patent holder does not submit the winning bid, the patent holder would agree to issue a voluntary license to the winner, waive the right to litigate for patent infringement in the specific circumstance, or match the winning bid. In all cases, a winning generics supplier would be required to pay a reasonable royalty to the patent holder, so that the cost advantage of the generics supplier would have to be sufficient to cover the royalty rate. Such a best-price-wins procedure could be established as part of the voluntary pricing guidelines for the group of low-income countries, and in conjunction with the obligations on the donors and recipient countries.

In any case, voluntary arrangements need to be backed by safeguards in case the voluntary arrangements prove difficult to implement. Safeguards are even more essential, of course, in the unlikely case that no voluntary guidelines can be approved at all. Assuming that a patent holder chooses neither to offer an essential medicine on a no-profit basis nor to license the medicine to a generics producer, the low-income country will still need a way to ensure access at low cost. The current rules on intellectual property rights in the world trading system, known as *TRIPS* (trade-related intellectual property rights), envisage compulsory licensing as such a safeguard. Under compulsory licensing, a national authority assigns to a local producer the right to produce a patented product, and the local producer must pay fair compensation (in the form of a royalty) to the patent holder. Compulsory licensing is useful for the small group of developing countries (such as Brazil, India, and South Africa) that have a high-quality generics sector with the know-how[121] and capacity to produce for the home market.

For low-income countries without local production capacity, however, compulsory licensing is of little practical value by itself.[122] The Commission therefore recommends that, for such countries, compulsory licensing should be interpreted broadly to cover imports from a low-cost producer in a third country. For example, low-income sub-Saharan African countries would, in an emergency (and in the absence of voluntary arrangements), be able to invoke a compulsory license to allow third countries to supply low-income countries with essential medicines from a manufacturer based, say, in South Africa or India, even if that producer does not hold the patent and is under patent restrictions in its own home-country market. As always, the producer would be required to pay a reasonable royalty to the patent holder, and the production would be directed only for use within the country invoking the compulsory license. The country invoking the safeguard would be bound not to permit the production to be diverted into the international markets.

The specific suggestions that we have offered here can be combined with other more standard approaches to ensure competitive tendering. These include bulk purchasing arrangements, transparency in pricing (including posted price lists for key drugs, as the industry has begun to announce in the case of antiretrovirals), and ad hoc negotiations over licenses for particular products. The Commission feels that a voluntary pricing and licensing approach, backed by strong protection for intellectual property rights in the higher-income markets to preserve the incentives for R&D, as well as safeguards and other standard tendering devices, could prove a workable and effective solution for all major stakeholders. In these circumstances, it would be our hope and expectation that safeguards such as compulsory licenses would remain little used in practice. In the event that such voluntary guidelines cannot be worked out, however, the Commission believes that the international trade rules regarding access to essential medicines should be applied in a manner that gives priority to health needs of the poor. This could mean a very expansive use of compulsory licensing by developing countries to promote active competition by high-quality generics producers, or even a delay in application of TRIPS beyond 2005/2006 in the low-income countries if no better alternatives are present.

The bottom line is clear: the best solution is a cooperative and voluntary arrangement that would protect intellectual property rights to the maximum extent while ensuring access of the poor to essential medicines at the lowest possible prices through various mechanisms of differential pricing.

The Scale of Donor Assistance

To estimate global donor needs, we began with targets for scaling up the coverage of essential interventions, and then made estimates of the incremental costs of shifting from the current levels of coverage to the target levels within each country. The methodology and results are summarized in Appendix 2, and elaborated in the Background Paper on costs of Working Group 5. Adding up all of the interventions, and including the costs of system strengthening such as substantial additional training, management and supervision, and the costs of ensuring increased quality (such as increased health-worker pay to ensure better motivation and performance), we arrived at a total cost per country. Since the scaling up is assumed to take time, we estimated the increased annual costs as of 2007 and 2015. We then estimated the increase in domestic resource mobilization that each country could achieve, assuming that each country would mobilize an additional 1 percent of GNP of budgetary revenues for health by 2007 and 2 percent of budgetary revenues by 2015. We then took the difference of the costs and the increased revenues, and designated this as the "net financing gap" to be covered by donor assistance at country level.

This amount is the gap for country-level programs. There are additional expenses regarding global public goods as well, especially R&D and the operations of international health institutions, mainly the WHO.

The estimated gap for all country-level programs is shown in Table A2.6 to be around $22 billion per year in 2007 (of which $14 billion would be directed at least-developed countries, $6 billion would be directed at other low income countries, and $2 billion for low-middle-income countries). Another $3 billion or so would be needed for increased R&D outlays directed at biomedical and health research for low-income countries, and $2 billion for the supply of other global public goods. The total donor assistance would then be $27 billion per year by the year 2007. This would increase to $38 billion in 2015, as coverage is extended and especially as the number of people receiving AIDS treatment continues to rise. Official development assistance for health would be around 0.1 percent of donor GNP, or one penny of aid for every $10 of donor GNP. These calculations assume, of course, that the recipient countries undertake strong domestic measures to justify and make effective use of the large increase in donor support. Without those domestic measures, actual aid disbursements would fall short of the numbers shown in the table.

The implication is that considerably more donor financing will be needed to achieve broad coverage of essential health interventions. But the numbers, while big in absolute terms, are manageable. Total donor-country GNP is around $25 trillion per year (2001). Total official development assistance (ODA) is around $53 billion, or 0.2 percent of GNP of the donor nations (Table 13). Five donor countries subscribe to the international standard of 0.7 percent of GNP, and Ireland and the United Kingdom are committed to raising their ODA to that level. The heads of the IMF, World Bank, and many other donor agencies have recently endorsed that standard once again. If all donors were to raise their ODA to 0.7 percent of their GNP, the total ODA would be around $175 billion per year today and $200 billion by 2007.[123] This would clearly be sufficient to accommodate health assistance of some $27 billion, plus significant and warranted increases in other areas of ODA as well, especially education, water and sanitation, environmental management, and other urgent areas for poverty reduction and economic growth. We stress this point because we do not believe that ODA for health should come at the expense of ODA in other critical areas such as education. It is fair to say, indeed, that other priority areas for social investment (education, environmental management) should also put in a claim for increased ODA. A

Table 13. AID TO ALL RECIPIENT COUNTRIES AND TO LEAST-DEVELOPED COUNTRIES, 1999 (percent of donor-country GNP)

Country	Aid to All Recipient Countries, percent of GNP	Aid to Least-Developed Countries, percent of GNP
Australia	0.26	0.05
Austria	0.25	0.04
Belgium	0.30	0.07
Canada	0.28	0.05
Denmark	1.00	0.32
Finland	0.33	0.08
France	0.39	0.06
Germany	0.26	0.05
Greece	0.16	0.00
Ireland	0.32	0.12
Italy	0.15	0.03
Japan	0.34	0.06
Luxembourg	0.66	0.16
Netherlands	0.79	0.16
New Zealand	0.27	0.06
Norway	0.91	0.30
Portugal	0.26	0.12
Spain	0.23	0.03
Sweden	0.70	0.17
Switzerland	0.35	0.10
United Kingdom	0.23	0.05
United States	0.10	0.02
All Donors	0.24	0.05

Source: Calculated from Tables 31 and 39, 2000 Development Cooperation Report, Organisation for Economic Cooperation and Development, Paris.

significant increase of ODA for the health sector should not and need not be prejudicial to other valid claims for increased assistance. We are stressing the urgent need of ODA for health, not the case for ODA in place of other targets of assistance.

It is important to realize just how small donor financing for health has been relative to the size of the donor economies and the recipient country needs. Table 14 shows the annual flows of bilateral donor support

Table 14. Official Development Assistance for Health and Population
Programs, Bilateral Sources, by Agency (US $ millions)
(Average 1997–1999)

Country	Health	Population	Total	% of GNP
United States[1]	535.8	385	920.8	0.012
Japan	338.6	21.2	359.9	0.009
United Kingdom[2]	267	19.3	286.3	0.023
France	184.4	1.5	185.9	0.013
Germany	118.6	65.7	184.3	0.009
Netherlands	80	21.5	101.4	0.026
Australia	64.8	14.9	79.6	0.021
Sweden	58.7	20.4	79.1	0.035
Spain	72.9	1.9	74.8	0.014
Belgium	58.8	1.7	60.5	0.024
Norway	41.3	15.1	56.4	0.037
Denmark	48.1	0.9	49	0.028
Austria	48.9	0.1	49	0.023
Canada	22.6	6.1	28.7	0.005
Italy	20.6	1	21.6	0.002
Switzerland	17.2	0.7	17.9	0.006
Finland	16	1.2	17.2	0.014
Luxembourg	16.2	0.5	16.7	0.089
Ireland	10.4	—	10.4	0.015
Portugal	8.6	0.1	8.7	0.008
Greece	5.8	—	5.8	0.005
New Zealand	3.1	0.2	3.3	0.006
Total[3]	1,982.4	577.5	2,559.8	0.011

Notes: (1) Source: USAID database, covers all accounts
       (2) Source DFID database
       (3) All other bilaterals: from DAC online database

for health, on average, for 1997 to 1999. Total bilateral flows averaged
$2.55 billion, which represented just 0.01 percent of donor GNP. That
comes to one penny per every $100 of donor GNP! Table 15 shows devel-
opment assistance targeted at specific diseases. AIDS programs received
commitments of just $287 million per year on average during 1997 to
1999, with less than half of that going to Africa.[124] Malaria was funded
at $87 million and tuberculosis at just $81 million. Since these numbers

Table 15. DEVELOPMENT ASSISTANCE TO HEALTH FOR SPECIFIC DISEASE CONTROL: ANNUAL AVERAGE COMMITMENTS, 1997–1999, SELECTED BILATERAL AND MULTILATERAL AGENCIES ($US millions)

	Total	World Bank	IDB	AfDB	WHO	UNICEF	DFID	USAID
Total	1,743	504	23	2	0	322	209	209
AIDS	287	145	NA	0	0	25	7	17
Vaccine-Preventable Childhood Diseases	251	17	NA		0	104	110	0
Malaria	87	62	NA		0	25	0	0
Tuberculosis	81	58	NA		0	17	1	5

Source: Data provided by AfDB, IADB, WB, WHO, UNICEF, DFID, and USAID.

represent the amounts specifically earmarked for these diseases, it is likely that additional unearmarked funds also went to fight these diseases. Still, the conclusion is inescapable that donor support has been very modest compared both to donor capacity and the extent of need.

Private philanthropy by individuals, foundations, and corporations can also play an increased role. The single most significant contribution to global health in recent years has been the donation of more than $20 billion of personal wealth by Bill and Melinda Gates to establish the Gates Foundation. This foundation now contributes nearly $1 billion per year to global health initiatives. In the 20th century, the Rockefeller Foundation played a similar, pivotal role in global public health. Corporate philanthropy is also needed. As we noted earlier, several pharmaceutical companies have donated medicines to low-income countries, and these donations have become the centerpiece of important global public-private partnerships for disease control, in areas including lymphatic filariasis, African trypanosomiasis, leprosy, malaria, onchocerciasis, trachoma, mother-to-child transmission of AIDS, control of fungal infections in HIV/AIDS, tetanus, and guinea-worm disease.

Finally, we stress that the $27 billion per year estimate is based on a normative target for scaling up health interventions. With a bold international program, we believe that most countries can be inspired and supported to join this effort. In some countries, though, weak national leadership or implementation capacity may fail to seize the opportunity for improved health services, or weak implementation capacity may mean that proposals are not convincing. The capacity to use ODA effectively would thereby be diminished. We interpret the $27 billion per year therefore as an upper limit of what is likely to be usable in the next few years. Such sums must be available for the circumstance that most low-income countries organize their own efforts to make effective use of large-scale aid; a lack of donor assistance should not be the limiting factor in scaling up, as has too often been the case in the past. Still, it is unlikely that all such funds would actually be drawn.

Middle-income countries generally have the means to ensure universal coverage of essential interventions out of their domestic resources, except in the case of a few high-prevalence HIV/AIDS countries. Nonetheless, in scaling up health coverage, many middle-income countries will find it convenient to obtain international loan financing and advisory assistance. We recommend that the World Bank and the regional development banks stand prepared to offer adequate non-concessional loan assistance for the health sector for these countries. Such non-concessional loans—extended by the International Bank for Reconstruction and Development (IBRD) at the cost of funds—is not counted as ODA.

Despite the seeming odds, we are optimistic that the needed resources can indeed be mobilized. The Commission found evidence of rising donor assistance for health in recent years, both in absolute dollar terms and as a proportion of overall development assistance. Governments and their citizens are increasingly aware of the universal threat posed by infectious diseases and the inability of individual nations to protect their borders against the importation of diseases, including drug-resistant forms, and disease vectors. The world's increased mobility and interconnectedness mean that an outbreak or epidemic is a much wider potential threat. Moreover, international public health crises, particularly the HIV/AIDS pandemic and resurgent growth in TB and malaria, are receiving increased attention at all levels of policy makers, and international health issues are increasingly a matter of public debate in the media and popular press. There is a growing consensus on the centrality of health objectives to local, national, and global development, and new ideas and resources are entering the health sector from private philanthropy as well as the private commercial sector. The focus on issues of effective implementation throughout this Report should provide assurance that funds will not be used where they are not needed (bearing in mind the need, though, not to abandon countries facing complex emergencies or other crises). Current debates on the costs and benefits of globalization further contribute to these growing concerns over health, and are giving insistence to the concept of GPGs in the heath sector. Progress on debt relief has also drawn increased national and international attention to the challenges and opportunities for improved performance in the health sector.

New Approaches to Donor–Recipient Relations

Citizens in the rich countries will be vastly more prepared to support a large increase in donor funding for health if they are confident that the programs will work. A perceived lack of effectiveness is surely the greatest reason for public dislike of aid projects. Special care, therefore, is needed to raise standards for use of donor funding, and to demonstrate success or failure of donor programs. We therefore underscore the following consideration as key to the scaling up of donor support:

Clear and quantifiable targets for coverage of health interventions and for health outcomes

Selectivity in donor support to those countries that are helping themselves

Transparency in the design, implementation, and evaluation of programs

Inputs to donor-supported programs from accredited experts

Independent review, and cutoff in funding to governments that fail to perform according to commitments

Fortunately, a new donor–recipient architecture is already being put in place as part of the increased attention to support of country-led poverty reduction strategies. For the low-income countries, this has been formalized in the Poverty Reduction Strategy Paper (PRSP).

Meeting these goals will require not only the good will of donors and recipient countries, but also new modalities for actually delivering the funding. We believe that recent innovations in donor-supported global health are promising and should be extended. The Sector-Wide Approaches (SWAps) to health-sector scaling up have given donors and recipient countries a new tool for bold and coordinated actions. The Multi-Country AIDS Program of the World Bank has permitted a substantial increase in concessional financing for AIDS in Africa during 2001, and there is no reason why the Bank could not substantially further increase its financing for health, especially if the Bank's Board consents to the allocation of funding in the form of grants rather than loans, a step that we respectfully recommend as realistic given the needs of the recipient countries. The new Global Alliance for Vaccines and Immunizations (GAVI), backed by a substantial donation of the Bill and Melinda Gates Foundation, has shown how a pool of international funds can stimulate country-level leadership in scaling up health interventions (in this case, immunizations).

The SWAp was developed during the mid-1990s as a means for addressing many of the delivery programs of donor-supported programs. The basic idea of the SWAp is that the donors work together with national authorities, agreeing on strategies for support, and seeking ways to pool their assistance for a country-designed and country-led strategy. The support is negotiated at the country level (usually as part of the Consultative Group process of donors). The success of the SWAp, at the country level, depends on the extent to which national governments and donors are able to subscribe to, support, and then sustain a collaborative mechanism for assistance to the health sector. They are best suited to countries that have commitment to, and at least moderate capacity for, implementing pro-poor health programs. While some commentators have concluded that the SWAp has not introduced novel features—such as resource pooling—in most countries, those who work at the country level point to numerous examples of the approach improving the synergy and effectiveness of development assistance for health. The use of the SWAp has limited the inevitable tendency for those who provide finance to expect to determine how their funds are used and to get credit for that use.

The new Global Fund to Fight AIDS, Tuberculosis, and Malaria (GFATM) can similarly provide substantial international funding for HIV/AIDS, malaria, and TB. We endorse the key concepts that have gone into the design of the GFATM: country-led processes, measurable results, and public and private funding.[125] Additional and complementary pools of funds at country level will be needed for other areas of health, and for overall health-system strengthening. Assuming, as we believe likely, that GAVI and the GFATM live up to their great promise, additional pools of donor funds could be mobilized for health-sector strengthening, childhood illnesses, and other priority areas for scaling up. One realistic option would be to expand the scope of the GFATM to disburse funding for a wider range of concerns beyond HIV/AIDS, TB, and malaria.

In the Commission's view, the GFATM should work according to the following broad principles:

It should provide large-scale financing only for those countries that have prepared viable strategies.

It should offer small grants at the outset to enable relevant institutions within each country to prepare proposals for submission to the GFATM.

It should encourage country proposals to reflect a national dialogue on health delivery that engages all major stakeholders, perhaps through the National Commission on Macroeconomics and Health which we advocate.

It should target its financial assistance to those countries that face a financing gap. The predominant flows should therefore be directed at the low-income countries, especially the least-developed countries, and in the form of grants rather than loans.[126] Middle-income countries (aside from a few high HIV/AIDS prevalence countries) should seek external financing from the World Bank and the regional development banks rather than from the GFATM.

It should encourage demonstrated fiscal effort on the part of recipient countries, along the lines suggested in this Report.

It should operate on principles of outcomes-based performance standards, transparency, and ex post auditing and evaluation. Countries that fail to deliver on previous commitments would face reduced access to donor assistance.

It should take a hard line on corrupt use of donor funds, which should jeopardize country access to future funding.

It should operate according to independent expert evaluations of country proposals, with projects being evaluated according to epidemiological needs, feasibility, cost effectiveness, and operational monitorability. Realistic budgets for these purposes will need to be incorporated into the operation of donor-supported projects.

It should devote a substantial amount of its annual funding, perhaps 5 percent of each country's funding, for operational research.

In fact, these principles and approaches for the Global Fund are similar to those that guide the GAVI, the very important public-private partnership for expanded immunization coverage in poor countries that has been underwritten primarily by the Gates Foundation.[127] GAVI is an attractive working model for the new Global Fund to Fight AIDS, Tuberculosis, and Malaria. Key aspects of GAVI operations worth noting include: country eligibility based upon a coherent multi-year plan presented by the country; external review of proposals by independent experts;

specific and monitorable performance criteria (e.g., number of immunizations delivered); and incentive-payment mechanisms (for example, half of the payment from GAVI is made up front, and the other half is made upon demonstration that the immunization has been carried out).

The world's multilateral agencies, especially the World Health Organization and the World Bank, should have special and intensified responsibilities in the new global architecture. One hundred and ninety-one countries are the Member States that govern WHO: the Secretariat, in responding to the mandates of these Member States, is the legitimate inter-governmental authority on global health matters. Generous voluntary finance supplements the assessed contributions to the WHO budget, and has enabled the organization to establish a widespread network of more than 100 country teams, six regional offices, collaborating centers, and headquarters in Geneva. This capacity has been developed, over the years, as a respected locus of authoritative evidence on approaches to disease control, the development of health systems so that they respond equitably to people's priorities, and the promotion of public health. WHO is the multilateral agency, above all others, that can mobilize global expertise, drawing upon national-level institutions in the donor countries (such as the NIH in the United States), in recipient countries (such as the Center for Health and Population Research in Bangladesh, formerly ICDDR,B), and leaders from academia, the private sector, and those concerned with the delivery of health services. The WHO should provide a technical secretariat for the Global Fund to Fight AIDS, Tuberculosis, and Malaria and build up the capacity of its country teams so that they can better support the application of the sector-wide approach to national or local-level health action. This involvement of WHO would ensure the professionalism and expertise needed for success in donor-supported programs. The WHO will also have a special role to play in establishing the evidence base for a greatly increased disease control effort, including the epidemiological baselines that will be necessary for effective scaling up of health system action in each country.

This enhanced role for WHO will require reforms and improvements. In particular, the Member States should permit the WHO Secretariat to work in more flexible partnerships with other institutions (concerns expressed in the WHO Executive Board and the World Health Assembly about the potential for conflict of interest have constrained this more open way of working). The management and accountability of regional and country-level operations should be strengthened. Given tight budget constraints, greater prioritization and focus will be required, but the budget squeeze itself should also be eased, in line with overall increased provision of global public goods.

The World Bank is unique in its capacity to link the health sector to the broader development agenda. Health, we have stressed, is a central part of the overall development agenda, but it is just one part of a much larger effort. The World Bank is the global institution most qualified to assist countries and the international community in linking health interventions to other aspects of the development agenda. In recent years, the Bank has been a major provider of development assistance for health, yet the Bank's own efforts in public health are now hampered by its limited capacity to make grants rather than loans for health-related projects in the low-income countries.[128] We therefore endorse the increased reliance on grants for the low-income countries. At the same time, developed countries should increase their commitments and long-term contributions to International Development Assistance (IDA) to allow the Bank to scale up its grant programs as needed.[129] In addition, the IBRD and the regional development banks should enlarge the amount of non-concessional assistance that the Bank offers to its middle-income Member States. The World Bank should also consider expanding its support of global public goods in health, such as grants to TDR, IRV, and HRP, through increasing its health-related partnerships under the Bank's Development Grant Facility.

Absorbing Increased Donor Flows
The question arises as to whether a large increase in donor aid to the health sector could be destabilizing, either in macroeconomic terms or on a sectoral level. An analogy is sometimes made to the "Dutch Disease" phenomenon, in which a resource boom (usually a commodity discovery or rise in world commodity prices) gives rise to domestic inflation, an overvalued exchange rate, and a squeeze on traditional exports. Could the same occur with a large infusion of donor assistance to the health sector?

In our view, the macroeconomic magnitudes are generally not worrisome, though in cases where the aid is a large proportion of GNP, care must be taken to accommodate the increases into the macroeconomic policy framework. In total, for the least-developed countries, incremental donor assistance would be on the order of 6 percent of GNP, though reaching 8 percent in the low-income sub-Saharan African countries. For other low-income countries, the share of GDP would be much smaller (perhaps 1 percent of GNP). Unlike a commodity boom, assistance would be built up gradually over time and then sustained for a decade or more. Moreover, half of this amount or more would fall on tradable goods, especially drugs and diagnostics, and so would not unduly or abruptly raise demand for domestic goods. We might guess, therefore, that the rise in demand for nontradeable output in the health sector would probably be on the order of 3 percent of GNP. Since all of this would be externally financed, there would be no problem with a growing budget deficit or money creation. We should note that, for many poor developing countries, donor assistance as a percent of GNP is vastly larger than the sums that we are discussing. In 1999, net official development assistance for Malawi constituted 24.6 percent of GNP, for the United Republic of Tanzania 11.3 percent of GNP, for Senegal 11.2 percent of GNP, and for Uganda 9.2 percent of GNP. All of these countries were macroeconomically stable, with at least modest economic growth and fairly low inflation.

The bigger issue, by far, will be the capacity of the health sector itself to absorb the increased flows. As a percent of domestic output, the value added originating in the health sector would rise from just a couple of percent of the gross domestic product (GDP) to perhaps 6 percent or more of the GDP.[130] As discussed elsewhere in this report, in many countries this raises issues of the quality of public administration and governance. In all countries, this will require greatly expanded implementation capacity, including management systems and strengthened local management expertise, and in many cases new systems of accountability both downward to the community level and upward to the central level. Moreover, we are assuming a substantial rise in wages of public sector health workers, to attract and retain staff and ensure good motivation and performance. This could, however, prove politically difficult to manage because of wage demands in other parts of the public sector. The wage increase is necessary, in fact, to slow, let alone reverse, the brain drain of professionals that is afflicting the health sectors of the low-income countries, and to ensure that lower-level workers have salaries they can live on, but it will still require political skill to manage.[131] There needs to be a judicious phase-in period, coupled with aggressive efforts to train new health sector workers, and to shift as much basic health provision as possible to paramedical workers who can be more rapidly trained and who are less internationally mobile. There are steps that can be taken to help avoid the rigidities of pay scales and terms of service associated with central government rules and regulations. These include decentralization of public management to units with greater autonomy, raising allowances and other terms of service rather than salaries per se, and greater use of private-sector and NGO providers. There will be problems, in other words, but they will be ameliorated by a medium-term program for scaling up, one which anticipates many of the challenges ahead.

THE MACROECONOMIC BENEFITS OF SCALING UP

A massive scaling up of essential health interventions should lead to a significant reduction in the burden of disease in low-income countries. The best estimate of the combined effect of the interventions that we recommend would be to reduce total deaths in the developing world due to infectious diseases and maternal conditions by around 8 million per year by 2015, which would be associated with a reduction of around 330 million DALYs. The reduction in deaths is shown by comparing Table 16a (baseline) and 16b (with scaled-up interventions), and the associated reduction in DALYs is shown by comparing Table 17a (baseline) and 17b (with scaled-up interventions).

Most, though not all, of these deaths would be saved in the low-income countries; some would be saved in the middle-income countries. At this stage we could not make separate epidemiological estimates for the two groups because we don't have an appropriate epidemiological baseline for each country. Indeed, our estimates will require signifcant refinement in the future based on more detailed epidemioligical data and modeling.

If we take the most conservative assumption that each DALY is valued at one year of average per capita income, and that per capita income in the low-income countries is likely to be around $563 per capita in 2015 (assuming 2 percent growth per year during 2000–2015), an extremely conservative estimate of direct economic savings would be 330 million DALYs × $563 / DALY, or $186 billion per year as of 2015. More conventionally, each DALY would be valued at a multiple of annual income, perhaps three times current income, in which case the direct benefits would exceed $500 billion per year. Even with the very conservative assumption, the direct benefits are nearly three times the costs of scaling up in the low-income countries, which we estimate to be around $66 billion.

The actual benefits could be much larger than this if the benefits of improved health help to spur economic growth, as we would expect. The improvements in life expectancy and reduced disease burden would tend to stimulate growth through the channels we have already discussed: faster demographic transition (to lower fertility rates), higher investments

Table 16a. UNDER-60 ANNUAL DEATHS FROM GROUP I, GROUP II, AND GROUP III CAUSES, WITHOUT INTERVENTIONS, WHO DEMOGRAPHICALLY DEVELOPING REGIONS, 1998–2020

	1998	2005	2010	2015	2020
Group I*	13,956,966	13,547,795	13,255,530	12,963,265	12,671,000
Infectious and Nutritional Deficiencies	9,073,058	8,974,403	8,903,935	8,833,468	8,763,000
Maternal Conditions	491,185	415,081	360,720	306,360	252,000
Respiratory Infections	2,290,921	2,223,810	2,175,873	2,127,937	2,080,000
Perinatal Conditions	2,101,802	1,934,502	1,815,001	1,695,501	1,576,000
Group II*	7,809,835	9,347,660	10,446,107	11,544,553	12,643,000
Malignant Neoplasm	2,242,159	2,814,836	3,223,890	3,632,945	4,042,000
Cardiovascular Diseases	2,975,450	3,547,716	3,956,477	4,365,239	4,774,000
Others	2,592,226	2,985,109	3,265,739	3,546,370	3,827,000
Group III*	4,578,256	5,044,311	5,377,207	5,710,104	6,043,000

*Groups I, II, and III are defined in detail in the World Health Report 2000, Annex Table 4, pp. 170–175.

Table 16b. UNDER-60 AANNUAL DEATHS FROM GROUP I, GROUP II, AND GROUP III CAUSES, WITH INTERVENTIONS, WHO DEMOGRAPHICALLY DEVELOPING REGIONS, 1998–2020

	1998	2005	2010	2015	2020
Group I*	13,956,966	9,868,714	5,155,625	4,727,703	4,593,479
Infectious and Nutritional Deficiencies	9,073,058	6,489,866	2,849,259	2,826,710	2,804,160
Maternal Conditions	491,185	234,334	203,645	106,253	87,400
Respiratory Infections	2,290,921	1,664,462	718,038	702,219	686,400
Perinatal Conditions	2,101,802	1,475,851	1,384,682	1,092,521	1,015,519
Group II*	7,809,835	8,132,367	9,088,004	9,293,184	10,177,417
Malignant Neoplasm	2,242,159	2,198,138	2,517,573	2,439,041	2,713,667
Cardiovascular Diseases	2,975,450	2,984,297	3,328,143	3,325,363	3,636,750
Others	2,592,226	2,949,932	3,242,288	3,528,780	3,827,000
Group III*	4,578,256	5,044,311	5,377,207	5,710,104	6,043,000

*Groups I, II, and III are defined in detail in the World Health Report 2000, Annex Table 4, pp. 170–175.

Table 17a. UNDER-60 ANNUAL DALYs FROM GROUP I, GROUP II, AND GROUP III CAUSES, WITHOUT INTERVENTIONS, WHO DEMOGRAPHICALLY DEVELOPING REGIONS, 1998–2020

	1998	2005	2010	2015	2020
Group I*	458,011,800	460,221,000	461,799,000	463,377,000	464,955,000
Infectious and Nutritional Deficiencies	296,833,900	303,295,250	307,910,500	312,525,750	317,141,000
Maternal Conditions	15,111,100	15,142,250	15,164,500	15,186,750	15,209,000
Respiratory Infections	78,881,900	76,813,750	75,336,500	73,859,250	72,382,000
Perinatal Conditions	67,184,900	64,969,750	63,387,500	61,805,250	60,223,000
Group II*	376,217,100	432,577,250	472,834,500	513,091,750	553,349,000
Malignant Neoplasm	43,768,600	54,984,000	62,995,000	71,006,000	79,017,000
Cardiovascular Diseases	64,775,300	77,738,250	86,997,500	96,256,750	105,516,000
Others	267,673,200	299,855,000	322,842,000	345,829,000	368,816,000
Group III*	197,612,600	216,174,500	229,433,000	242,691,500	255,950,000

*Groups I, II, and III are defined in detail in the World Health Report 2000, Annex Table 4, pp. 170–175.

Table 17b. Under-60 Annual DALYs from Group I, Group II, and Group III Causes, With Interventions, WHO Demographically Developing Regions, 1998–2020

	1998	2005	2010	2015	2020
Group I*	458,011,800	335,241,967	124,980,732	125,580,567	126,474,099
Infectious and Nutritional Deficiencies	296,833,900	219,328,853	98,531,360	100,008,240	101,485,120
Maternal Conditions	15,111,100	8,548,561	203,645	106,253	87,400
Respiratory Infections	78,881,900	57,493,044	24,861,045	24,373,553	23,886,060
Perinatal Conditions	67,184,900	49,566,073	1,384,682	1,092,521	1,015,519
Group II*	376,217,100	376,337,684	411,361,070	413,030,810	445,437,265
Malignant Neoplasm	43,768,600	42,937,640	49,193,522	47,671,107	53,049,431
Cardiovascular Diseases	64,775,300	65,392,513	73,181,286	73,326,715	80,380,250
Others	267,673,200	268,007,531	288,986,261	292,032,988	312,007,584
Group III*	197,612,600	216,174,500	229,433,000	242,691,500	255,950,000

*Groups I, II, and III are defined in detail in the World Health Report 2000, Annex Table 4, pp. 170–175.

in human capital, increased household saving, increased foreign investment, and greater social and macroeconomic stability. Because we lack
adequate epidemiological baselines, we cannot precisely translate the lives
saved into increased years of life expectancy. Still, we can offer an illustration. If the improved health outcomes raise the life expectancy of the
low-income countries by one-half of the existing 19-year gap with the
high-income countries, say from 59 years to 68 years, the effect on economic growth would be around 0.5 percent per year. Additional growth
dividends would come from reducing the burden of malaria and
HIV/AIDS, which directly impede foreign investment. Even taking just the
0.5 percent per annum estimate, per capita income of the low-income
countries would be 10 percent higher than otherwise after 20 years. Since
the GNP of the low-income countries will be around $1.8 trillion in 2020,
the 10 percent gain would amount to $180 billion per year as of
2020.[132] Speaking very roughly, the annual gains from increased per capita growth are likely to be the same order of magnitude as the gains from
increased longevity (reduced DALYs). Combining the valuation of lives
saved plus faster economic growth suggests economic benefits of at least
$360 billion per year during 2015–2020, and possibly much larger.

NEXT STEPS
We call on the world to commit during the coming year to a bold scaling
up of essential health services. The new PRSP process is coming into place
and should be harnessed with urgency to turn our global commitments on
poverty reduction into action. We need coordinated steps by the low-
income countries, the donor countries, and the multilateral agencies.

The Low-Income Countries
The Commission recommends that every developing country begin to map
out a path to universal access for essential health services. The starting
point is for government and civil society together to identify the essential
services to be made universally available, based on epidemiological and
economic analysis and the perceived priorities of communities. Within the
PRSP process, we recommend that each country establish in 2002 a
National Commission on Macroeconomic and Health (NCMH), chaired
by the Ministers of Finance and Health, and including leading representatives of civil society, charged with this task.[133] During our own work we
have found that combining the energies, expertise, and mandates of

finance and health leaders is critical. The NCMH would have a limited mandate, aiming to conclude its work by the end of 2003.

The NCMH would be assigned the following tasks: (1) identify the priority areas for health interventions and the financing strategies to address those priorities; (2) designate a set of essential interventions to be made universally available to the entire population on the basis of public financing (with the requisite donor support); (3) initiate a multi-year program of health-system strengthening, focused on service delivery at the local level and including training, construction, and bolstering of infrastructure, and management development to enable the health sector to achieve universal coverage of essential interventions; (4) establish quantified targets for reductions in the burden of disease based on sound epidemiological modeling; (5) identify key health synergies with other sectors (e.g., education etc); and (6) ensure consistency of the strategy with the overall macroeconomic framework. The NCMH would work closely with the WHO and the World Bank in carrying out these tasks. The WHO would help each country to establish the epidemiological baseline, to identify essential interventions, and to set quantified targets. The World Bank would help especially in the planning of the multi-year strategy for scaling up, including the design of a medium-term financing strategy based on domestic and donor resources.

The Donor Countries

Donor countries would begin to mobilize annual commitments of donor health financing of around 0.1 percent of combined GNP (approximately $27 billion per year by 2007), to be scaled up in conjunction with country-level programs and increased provision of global public goods in health. Actual disbursements would depend, of course, on the low-income countries designing sound, credible, and monitorable strategies for scaling up essential health interventions. The WHO and the World Bank, backed by a steering group of donor and recipient countries, could be charged with the coordination of the massive, multi-year scaling up of donor assistance in health and the monitoring of donor commitments and disbursements. Key international forums (such as the IMF/World Bank meetings, the World Health Assembly, the UN Conference on Development Finance, and World Bank–sponsored Consultative Group meetings) should provide venues for specific commitments to scaling up of donor assistance for health.

International Agencies

The global strategy will require bolstering the operations of existing international institutions such as WHO as well as creating new institutions such as the GFATM for AIDS, malaria, and TB, and the GHRF for health research. The WHO has a crucial role to play in several areas, most importantly advising member governments on appropriate health strategies. For this, its on-the-ground capacity in member countries will need to be bolstered. In addition, WHO will be critical in establishing epidemiological baselines in each country and at the world level, which will be needed as critical inputs to global disease control efforts. The WHO and the World Bank together have a shared responsibility in the analysis and dissemination of best practices in health systems reform as well as in giving support for policy reforms to address existing resource imbalances in the health sector. Finally, the IMF will be important in assisting donors and recipient countries to take account of the scaling up process in the macroeconomic policy framework of low-income countries, particularly with respect to the absorption of additional international funding. In addition to the WHO and the World Bank, the new GFATM must become operational in 2002, with adequate financing to initiate a bold process of scaling up interventions against HIV/AIDS, malaria, and TB. Funding will have to begin at several billion dollars per year, with a target of $8 billion per year by 2007.

Fighting disease will be the truest test of our common capacity to forge a true global community. There is no excuse in today's world for millions of people to suffer and die each year for lack of $34 per person needed to cover essential health services. A just and far-sighted world will not let this tragedy continue. Leaders will follow their pledges of recent years with the actions needed to give dignity, hope, and life itself to the world's poorest and most vulnerable people. We know that this can be accomplished, and we are optimistic that, in the coming year, the world will throw its energies behind this vital and worthy task.

NOTES

1.   The classifications are those used by the Development Assistance Committee of the OECD. There are five categories: least-developed countries, or LDCs, the 48 lowest-development countries as catagorized by the United Nations; other low-income countries or OLICs (countries with less than $755 GNP per capita in 1999 that are not LDCs); lower middle-income countries; upper middle income countries; and high-income countries. In the costing exercise we refer to the countries in Table A2.B.

2. In much of the low-income world, the age-specific death rates of many NCDs are falling while absolute burdens are rising due to an aging population. Tobacco-related illnesses and deaths, however, are rising even on an age-specific basis.

3. As just one example, new mechanisms for improving access to essential drugs for communicable diseases are beginning to be applied to cover key NCDs such as diabetes, some forms of cancers, mental disorders, hypertension, and other NCD conditions, but much more needs to be done for both communicable diseases and NCDs.

4. United Nations Development Program, Table 8, p. 169.

5. United Nations Development Program, 2001, Feature 1.3, p. 23.

6. For many middle-income countries, our recommendation to raise an additional 1 percent of GNP in health by 2007 and 2 percent of GNP in health by 2015 would be more than enough to provide universal access to essential interventions. Those countries might therefore choose to raise less than that amount in added revenues for health, or more realistically, might choose to extend coverage beyond the essential interventions outlined in this Report to include various non-communicable diseases that represent a growing burden on health in view of the aging of their populations.

7. Operational research involves the investigation of health interventions in practice, including issues of patient adherence, toxicity, dosing, and modes and costs of delivery. The goal is to optimize the treatment regimen to local conditions, and to identify how best to integrate the regimen into existing services. The issue of operational research is typically neglected in country programs. We might distinguish two kinds of operational research. Clinical research involves the questions of treatment regimens, such as dosage and toxicity. Nonclinical operational research involves questions of logistics, financial management, cultural aspects of treatment regimens, and other nonclinical dimensions of health-service delivery.

8. Later in the Report we distinguish between three types of disease: Type I, which is incident in large numbers (or at least potentially so) in both rich and poor countries; Type II, which is incident mainly in poor countries, but with a significant number of cases in rich countries; and Type III, which is overwhelmingly or exclusively incident in poor countries. The need for special R&D stimulus applies mainly to Type II and Type III diseases.

9. One part of surveillance is real-time monitoring of epidemics, which now takes place through the WHO Global Outbreak Alert and Response Network, which interlinks 72 existing networks. Yet the absence of requisite laboratory and epidemiological capacity in many low-income countries is a weakness that requires prompt solution.

10. Donors have called upon low-income countries to prepare a Poverty Reduction Strategy Paper (PRSP), which is the basis for a sustained and comprehensive attack on poverty supported by donor funding and debt cancellation.

11. These results are summarized in IMF, "Debt Relief for Poor Countries (HIPC): What Has Been Achieved," August 2001, http://www.imf.org/external/np/exr/facts/povdebt.htm.

12. In addition, it is important emphasize appropriate approaches and technologies in these related areas. For example, emphasis on the education of girls has a particularly large effect on the health of the poor. Similarly, fuel-efficient stoves represent an appropriate technology that can prevent death from indoor air pollution as well as save energy.

13. Where there is a roughly equivalent broad-based group already set up, there may be no need to create another one, but rather to modify the existing structure to cover the necessary tasks. We do, however, stress the advantages of having joint direction by the finance and health ministers as a key to achieving scaling up of health services.

14. Millions more deaths per year would be averted by a dramatic reduction in cigarette smoking as well.

15. All instances of dollar figures in this Report refer to US dollars. All cost projections are in constant-price 2002 $US.

16. The middle-income sub-Saharan African countries are included especially because of their high HIV/AIDS prevalence, and therefore the high costs of providing essential health interventions.

17. This amounts to an extra 1 percent of GNP in 2007 and an extra 2 percent of GNP in 2015, though for some countries a smaller amount would be sufficient to cover the costs of scaling up.

18. The donors are assumed to cover whatever gap remains after the mobilization of at least 1 percent of GNP in 2007 and 2 percent of GNP in 2015. If those sums are sufficient (or more than sufficient) to cover the total costs of scaling up, then we assume that the donors contribute no funds.

19. We estimate that total official development assistance (ODA) for health is now approximately $6 billion per year, including $5 billion in country programs in the low- and middle-income countries, and approximately $1 billion on global public goods for health. In this $6 billion we are including support for the health system and specific disease control programs, but are not counting family planning, which would add another $600 million or so to the total if it were counted in the total. Despite an ardent effort of the Commission and Working Group 6, it is not possible to get a precise accounting of current donor assistance for health, since the funds are spent in a wide variety of ways and reporting inevitably involves lags, differences in coverage and definitions across donors, and important discrepancies between commitments and disbursements. In addition to ODA, which is comprised of grants and concessional loans, there are also nonconcessional (market-interest-rate) loans for health, mainly from the World Bank to middle-

income developing countries, of around $0.5 billion per year; and R&D spending on diseases of the poor that are financed outside of ODA budgets (most likely, the sums are far below $0.5 billion).

20. Although we have confidence in the general range of our cost estimates, we urge care not to overinterpret the detailed results by region or disease. Precise calculations of the costs of scaling up by country and disease category will have to wait for detailed country-by-country estimation in much greater detail than the Commission itself could undertake.

21. When an individual dies young or in the middle age, the death is associated with many lost years of life. Also, disease can cause disability for years before eventual death. For both these reasons, DALYs lost per year are a multiple of deaths per year.

22. Per capita income in the low-income countries is currently around $410 per person per year in 1999. With growth of per capita income equal to 2 percent per annum, this would be $563 per year in 2015. 330 million DALYs would therefore result in a gain of $186 billion. There are good reasons to value each DALY at a multiple of per capita income, however, so that the direct benefits could be twice or more $186 billion. These calculations do not, furthermore, take into account the effects of better health on faster economic growth.

23. Our analysis suggests that most middle-income countries can afford to fund essential services out of their own domestic resources, if they demonstrate political will. Donor aid is needed overwhelmingly for low-income countries, with the exception of some funding for middle-income countries with very high HIV/AIDS prevalence which otherwise could not afford a comprehensive HIV/AIDS control effort.

24. Many have asked the Commission what to do if the donor money is not made available—in essence, how to triage with less money. We are asked to prioritize millions of readily preventable deaths per year, since we have already narrowed our focus to a small number of conditions that have an enormous social burden and that have low-cost interventions that are at least partially effective. Not only is this kind of triaging ethically and politically beyond our capacity, but it is also exceedingly hard to do in sensible way. Those who hope for a simple answer, for example to focus on the cheap interventions (immunizations) while putting off the expensive interventions (higher-cost prevention programs and antiretroviral therapy needed to fight AIDS) to a later date, misjudge the practical choices we face. The AIDS pandemic will destroy African economic development unless controlled; to fight measles but not AIDS will not begin to meet Africa's human and economic needs. It would be wrong to go to the other extreme as well, and let the legitimate need to fight AIDS end up starving the cheaper interventions, so we advocate *both*. Moreover, the infrastructure developed to fight AIDS will support the infrastructure needed to fight measles, especially if strengthening such com-

plementarities is explicitly built into the AIDS control effort. It is vastly more fruitful to design and finance a comprehensive program that addresses many critical health needs than to pick and choose the apparently inexpensive items.

25. Presented by UNAIDS and WHO at the WHO International Consultative Meeting on Anti-Retroviral Therapy, Geneva, May 2001.

26. *Differential pricing* refers to charging different prices in different markets, which are kept separate by physical and regulatory barriers. In this case, differential pricing would involve charging the lowest viable commercial price in the low-income markets, and at the same time charging higher (often patent-protected) prices in the high-income markets.

27. The participants and terms of reference of these working groups are in the Appendix 1.

28. Sen stresses that certain substantive freedoms ("the liberty of political participation or the opportunity to receive basic education or health care") are "constituent components of development" (essentially, end goals) as well as contributors to economic progress. See Sen (1999), *Development as Freedom*, especially Introduction and Chapter 1.

29. See Amir Attaran, "Health as a Human Right," CMH Policy Memorandum No. 3, http://www.cid.harvard.edu.

30. *Health of the body is prosperity* (Hausa Proverb); *Health is great riches* (English Proverb); *Without Health, no Wealth* (Serbian Proverb); *Health comes before making a livelihood* (Yiddish Proverb). Wolfgang Meider, *Prentice-Hall Encyclopedia of World Proverbs*, New York: Prentice Hall, Inc.

31. We use the term *population health* to mean health status at the level of whole populations, as summarized by population measures such as life expectancy, infant and child mortality, and disability-adjusted life years (DALYs). Economic growth signifies a sustained rise in the per capita income of the country (typically measured as the Gross National Product (GNP) per capita adjusted for purchasing power parity). Economic development signifies a broad-based and sustained rise in the material conditions of a society, evidenced not only by GNP per capita but also by several dimensions of material life (housing, consumption, diversity of goods and services, and the like).

32. We salute many earlier analysts who stressed the importance of the health-to-development linkages. A notable example is a WHO study by Abel-Smith and Leiserson, *Poverty, Development and Health Policy* (1978, especially pp. 27–34), in which the authors draw linkages from health to development that are similar to those that we describe: the effects of diseases such as malaria, onchocerciasis, schistosomiasis, and trypanosomiasis on limiting the exploitation of tropical arable land; adverse effects on livestock breeding; reduced migration and trade; delayed transition to reduced fertility; less societal openness to new methods of cultivation; and reduced food production during epidemics. We can only concur

with the summary statement that "What is required is a unified approach to development to help millions of poor break out of the vicious circle of poverty, ignorance, and ill health that encloses them and has tended to perpetuate itself from generation to generation over the centuries" (p. 32).

33. R. W. Fogel, "New Findings on Secular Trends in Nutrition and Mortality: Some Implications for Population Theory" in M. R. Rosenzweig and O. Stark (eds), *Handbook of Population and Family Economics*, Vol. 1a, Amsterdam, Elsevier Science, 1997: 433–481.

34. D. R. Gwatkin, "Health Inequalities and the Health of the Poor: What Do We Know? What Can We Do?" *Bulletin of the World Health Organization*, 2000, 78 (1); and Gwatkin et al., "Socio-Economic Differences in Health, Nutrition and Population" (a series of reports on 44 developing countries), World Bank, 2001. See also S. Gupta, M. Verhoeven, and E. Tiongson, "Public Spending on Health Care and the Poor," IMF Working Paper, 2001, Table 1, for a compilation of the data of the 44 country studies in the World Bank project.

35. It is also true, as a general matter, that at any given IMR, poorer countries had faster growth rates than richer countries, a phenomenon in economic development known as *conditional convergence*. Conditional convergence reflects the fact that, for two similarly placed countries, the poorer country has more scope to absorb capital and technology from the global leaders, and thereby to grow more rapidly than richer countries. On the other hand, the poorer countries may have worse attributes (e.g., higher IMR) or worse policies, so that the tendency toward convergence is only "conditional" on these other factors, not absolute.

36. Formally, the annual growth rate in these models is written as a linear function of several variables, including the natural logarithm of LEB. The estimated coefficient on ln (LEB) is typically around 3.5. Since ln (77) = 4.34 and ln (49) = 3.89, the growth difference is given by $3.5 \times (4.34-3.89)$, which equals around 1.6 percent per year.

37. Although all of the studies mentioned in this paragraph attempt to separate the direct effects of health from a poor institutional, policy, and governance environment more generally, we recognize that further research with more refined data—often at the household, village, or regional (subnational) levels—will shed further light on the specific effects of health versus other social conditions that may be correlated with health.

38. Purchasing-power-parity-adjusted dollars are US dollars adjusted for the fact that the average dollar price of goods is different (generally lower) in poor countries than in the United States.

39. IMF, OECD, UN, The World Bank, 2000. *Progress Towards the International Development Goals: 2000 A Better World for All*, Washington, DC.

40. The basic goal regarding poverty is to "halve the proportion of people living in extreme poverty" between 1990 and 2015. Extreme poverty is defined as living on less than $1 per day (1993 PPP $US). A related poverty goal is to "halve the number of people suffering from hunger" between 1990 and 2015.

41. Roll Back Malaria, a joint undertaking of WHO, UNDP, UNICEF, and the World Bank, aims to halve the number of deaths due to malaria by 2010. Stop TB, a global partnership including WHO, the World Bank, and UNICEF, aims to reduce the disease burden (prevalence and deaths) by half as of 2010 compared with 2000.

42. The study was carried out by the "State Failure Task Force," established by the US Central Intelligence Agency in 1994. The task force gave formal definition to state failure (as a case of revolutionary war, ethnic war, genocides, or politicides, and adverse or disruptive regime changes), and counted all cases during 1957–1994 in countries of 500,000 population or more. One hundred and thirteen cases of state failure were identified. Of all explanatory variables that were examined, three were most significant: infant mortality rates; openness of the economy, in that greater economic linkages with the rest of the world diminish the chances of state failure; and democracy, with democratic countries showing less propensity to state failure than authoritarian regimes. See State Failure Task Force, "State Failure Task Force Report: Phase II Findings," in the *Environmental Change and Security Project Report* of the Woodrow Wilson Center, Issue 5, Summer 1999, 49–72.

43. "[V]irtually every case of U.S. military intervention abroad since 1960 has taken place in a developing country that had previously experienced a case of state failure" (J. Sachs, "The Strategic Significance of Global Inequality," *The Washington Quarterly*, Summer 2001, p. 191).

44. See National Intelligence Council, "The Global Infectious Disease Threat and Its Implications for the United States," (Washington, DC, January 2000), located at http://www.cia.gov/. This report notes that, "As a major hub of global travel, immigration, and commerce with wide-ranging interests and a large civilian and military presence overseas, the United States and its equities abroad will remain at risk from infectious diseases," including the fact that "infectious diseases are likely to slow socioeconomic development in the hardest-hit developing and former communist countries and regions. This will challenge democratic development and transitions and possibly contribute to humanitarian emergencies and civil conflicts." See also National Intelligence Council Report, "Global Trends 2015: A Dialogue with Non-Governmental Experts," December 2000, located at http://www.cia.gov/.

45. B. Korber et al., *Science* 288, 1789 (2000).

46. As Laver and Garman recently wrote, "A worldwide epidemic (pandemic) of type A influenza could occur any time. Such an event will be caused by a 'new' virus against which the human population has no immunity, and past experience indicates that this new virus will probably arise in China. With today's crowded conditions and rapid transportation, the epidemic is expected to reach every corner of the globe. Millions of people will become ill, and many will die." Graeme Laver and Elspeth Garman, "The Origin and Control of Pandemic Influenza," *Science*, Vol. 293, 7 September 2001, 1776–1777.

47. As just one of many examples, of 416 Tibetan refugees arriving in Canada in 1999, 5 had MDR-TB. Bonnie Henry et al., "M. Tuberculosis Outbreak in Tibetan Refugee Claimants in Canada," presented at the 5th Annual Meeting of the International Union Against TB and Lung Disease, North American Region, Vancouver, February 2000. (http://www.hc-sc.gc.ca/hpb/lcdc/survlnce/fetp).

48. See Chris F. Curtis, "The mass effect of widespread use of insecticide-treated bednets in a community," CMH Policy Memorandum, http://www.cid.harvard.edu/.

49. Human Development Report 2001, p. 23. Similarly, 48 percent of the developing world population is in countries that are lagging, far behind, or slipping, regarding the maternal mortality goals.

50. Avoidable disease, in the Commission's analysis, refers to the excessive morbidity and mortality in a society compared with the disease and mortality rates in a benchmark society. Specifically, we calculate the excess disease burden in the low-income countries in comparison with the morbidity and mortality patterns of nonsmokers in high-income countries.

51. In economic jargon, poor health is said to reduce the "utility" of the individual even if there is no change in the level of consumption of goods and services or in the life span of the individual.

52. Such large valuations have been used in the recent economics literature. See, for example, Cutler and Richardson (1997); Topel and Murphy (1999); Philipson and Soares (2001); and Becker, Philipson, and Soares (2001).

53. 34.6 DALYs times 2.1 million deaths equals 72 million DALYs.

54. Technically, the econometric model in Gallup and Sachs (2001) assumes that the growth rate of the economy $d(\ln y)/dt$ is equal to $-a\,M - b\,\ln y + c\,Z$, where $\ln y$ is the natural logarithm of per capita GNP, M measures the proportion of the population vulnerable to malaria (varying between 0 and 1.0), and Z are other determinants of growth. Empirical estimates put coefficient a at around 1.3, and coefficient b at around 2.0. This suggests that the short-run effect of malaria on growth is -1.3 percent per year, and the long-run effect is to reduce the level of per capita income by $\exp(-a/b) = \exp(-0.65) = 0.52$. That is, the per capita income of a malarious economy is only 52 percent of the per capita income of a non-malarious economy.

55. Gertler and Gruber (2001) estimate that 35 percent of the costs of serious illness are not insured by other sources available to households (in a study based on Indonesian data). They also find that the more severe the illness, the less households are able to insure. Households are able fully to insure the economic costs of illnesses that do not affect physical functioning, insure 71 percent of the costs resulting from illnesses that moderately limit an individual's ability to function physically, but only 38 percent of the costs from illnesses that severely limit physical functioning. Their findings imply that there are nontrivial costs to the Indonesian economy from incomplete insurance of even these very extreme health events.

56. The Barker Hypothesis maintains that intrauterine growth retardation is associated with adult illness, including cardiovascular conditions.

57. World Health Report 1999.

58. The TFR is, roughly, the average number of children per women during her reproductive lifetime, calculated on the basis of the age-specific fertility rates in the country at any one time. The IMR is the number of deaths under age 1 per 1,000 live births.

59. Fertility rates tend to be lower in urban areas for several reasons: children are not economic assets in the cities, as they are on the farm; housing costs are higher; the opportunity cost of the mother's time may be higher; and children are more likely to be in school, with the attendant costs of providing for their school supplies, fees, uniform, etc.

60. Since there are a rising number of workers per person, GNP per person tends to increase even if GNP per worker remains unchanged.

61. Even if new hires are as productive as old hires, the firm must still pay substantial costs for screening and sorting new workers.

62. Gallup and Sachs, 2001 (*American Journal of Tropical Medicine and Hygiene*. Special Supplement). The takeoff of growth in southern Europe follows shortly after the postwar control of malaria. In earlier decades, the region had lagged behind the growth of northern Europe.

63. *Economist* (2001): The worst way to lose talent. 8 February.

64. The list of least-developed countries is shown in Table A2.B.

65. These are (with estimated numbers of deaths per year in parentheses): polio (720), diphtheria (5,000), pertussis (346,000), measles (888,000), tetanus including neonatal (410,000), *Haemophilus influenzae* b, or Hib (400,000), hepatitis B (900,000), and yellow fever (30,000). See http://www.vaccinealliance.org/reference/globalimmchallenges.html.

66. While comparing mortality among smokers and nonsmokers in developing countries with that among only nonsmokers in rich countries, this analysis seems perhaps to exaggerate the avoidable mortality. However, there are known interven-

tions that can substantially reduce smoking, so it seems valid to use nonsmokers as the baseline in an attempt to delineate the maximum conceivable improvement. This choice, as it happens, has little effect on the estimates presented here, since we report the reduction of mortality only to, 2015 and the big reductions in tobacco-related illnesses would necessarily come much later.

67. *Eradication* refers to the utter elimination of a disease from the world. *Elimination* refers to a halt in transmission of an infectious organism from a defined area. In the case of elimination, there is continuing concern over the reintroduction of the disease from another region. (See Basch 1999, p. 456).

68. For a recent chronicle of those events, see Jonathan Tucker, *Scourge*, New York: Atlantic Monthly Press, 2001.

69. Smallpox vaccinations are no longer used. The same may be possible with polio, although this point is still debated.

70. *DOTS* refers to a treatment regimen for tuberculosis in which the patient is directly observed taking the anti-TB medications for at least the first 2 months of therapy, to raise adherence. *Short course* refers to a 6-to-8 month regimen using a combination of anti-TB drugs.

71. WHO, UNICEF, UNAIDS, World Bank, UNESCO, and UNFPA, *Health A Key to Prosperity: Success Stories in Developing Countries*, 2000, published by the World Health Organization.

72. Experience shows, moreover, that family planning services are most effective when they are a part of comprehensive programs for reproductive health, that include family planning, safe pregnancy and delivery, and the prevention and treatment of reproductive tract infections and sexually transmitted diseases.

73. Rapid population growth has multiple and complex effects on economic development. At the household level, investments per child in education and health are reduced when households have many children, that is, when fertility rates are high. At the societal level, rapid rural population growth in particular puts enormous stress on the physical environment (e.g., deforestation, as forests are cut for firewood and new farm land) and on food productivity as land-labor ratios in agriculture decline. Desperately poor peasants are then likely to crowd cities, leading to very high rates of urbanization, with additional adverse consequences in congestion and in declining urban capital per person (e.g., policing services, water and sanitation, etc).

74. The report *Contraceptive Practices and the Donor Gap*, by the Interim Working Group (IWG) on Reproductive Health Commodity Security, estimates a donor gap for contraceptives and logistics on the order of $210 million by 2015, and roughly $100 million by 2007 (see Figure 9, p. 9 of that report). The IWG is a collaborative effort of John Snow, Inc., Population Action International, Program for Appropriate Technology in Health, and the Wallace Global Fund.

75. In Bangladesh, as the infant mortality rate came down from around 140 per 1,000 live births in 1970 to around 70 per 1,000 live births in 1995, the total fertility rate fell sharply, from 7.0 in 1970 to just 3.4 in 1990 and 3.1 in 1995. As a result, population growth slowed markedly, from around 2.5 percent per year in 1970 to 1.5 percent per year in 1995. The government invested heavily in family planning services; important nongovernmental organizations, such as Grameen Bank and BRAC, contributed to improvements in the social conditions of poor women, which in turn contributed to reduced fertility rates. Economic changes, in particular the ongoing process of urbanization, and especially the enormous increase in employment of young women in the export-oriented ready-made-garment sector, also led to delayed marriages of women and reduced fertility rates within marriage.

76. Although there is a single class of virus, HIV, which causes AIDS, there is a significant degree of genetic variation in the virus within a population and especially across regions. These subtypes, or clades, may have different transmissibility, though the evidence is not clear on this point. Some virologists have suggested that HIV1 clade C, which is prevalent especially in southern and eastern Africa and the Horn of Africa, may be more transmissible, and therefore more likely to result in high levels of adult prevalence.

77. Of course the social returns of treatment go far beyond the income levels of the patients, when we take into account the benefits for children who would otherwise be orphaned, and the many other adverse social spillovers associated with the disease.

78. Sanjeev Gupta, Marijn Verhoeven, and Erwin Tiongson, "Public Spending on Health Care and the Poor," IMF Working Paper, 2001.

79. Because of lower prices and wages for "nontraded" goods and services, including salaries in the health sector, $30 to $45 per person in low-income countries is probably equivalent to at least $60 to $90 per year in a high-income setting. Thus, at purchasing-power-parity prices, as are used in some analyses, the minimum cost of the essential package would probably be above $80 per person per year, as we noted in the text.

80. The graph is shown in log scales, with the natural logarithm of per capita income in US dollars on the x-axis and the natural logarithm of total health spending in US dollars on the y-axis.

81. The estimate in the graph is that each 1 percent increase in income leads to a 1.15 percent increase in health spending. This means that health expenditures as a share of income are slightly higher for rich countries than for poorer countries. For the 44 poorest countries, with per capita income of $500 or less per year, health spending averages 4.0 percent of income. For the 21 richest countries, with per capita income of $20,000 or more per year, health spending averages 6.5 percent of GNP.

82. See Fang Jing and Xiong Qiongfen, "Financial Reform and Its Impact on Health Service in Poor Rural China," presented at the Conference on Financial Sector Reform in China, Harvard University, September 2001. They write: "Due to the serious financial constraint, health facilities in poor counties have to rely on clinic services to earn their salaries, preventative care is largely ignored...Another result of the emphasis on curative services is the rapidly increasing medical expenditure and drug abuse" (pp. 13–14). Misra, Chaterjee, and Rao (2001) describe the burgeoning of unqualified, rural medical practitioners. "The estimated one million illegal practitioners are said to be managing 50–70% of primary consultations..." They note that "the technical quality of the care provided in the private sector is often poor—ranging from poor infrastructure to inappropriate and unethical treatment practices, to overprovision of services and exorbitant costs."

83. See Yuanli Liu and William Hsiao, "China's Poor and Poor Policy: The Case for Rural Health Insurance," presented at the Conference on Financial Sector Reform in China, Harvard University, 13 September 2001. Liu and Hsiao, using China's 1998 National Health Services Survey data, found that among all the rural households living in poverty that year, 44.3 percent of these household fell into poverty due to medical spending.

84. Without proposing a false precision on such a complex topic, it would plausible to suggest that a well-run government of a low-income country allocate total revenues in something the following manner: total revenues, 16 percent of GNP, of which: health, 4 percent; education, 5 percent; public administration, 2 percent; police and defense, 2 percent; public investments (infrastructure), 2 percent; and debt service, 1 percent. Of course, expenditures don't look much like this. Debt servicing payments are much higher, as are defense outlays in some countries. Education and health spending are considerably lower.

85. A summary of the voluminous literature on users fees, with widespread documentation of the fact that the poor tend to be priced out of the market for essential services, is provided by Dyna Ahrin-Tenkorang in *Mobilizing Resources for Health: The Case for User Fees Revisited*, CMH Paper No. WG3: 6, 2000. A recent paper, "The Bitterest Pill of All: The Collapse of Africa's Health Care System," Save the Children UK, May 2001, provides evidence and references that point to the same conclusion.

86. For the first 22 countries in the HIPC process, debt service savings from traditional and HIPC debt relief will be around 1.9 percent of GNP each year (p. 8, IMF 2001). For these countries, around 40 percent of the savings are being directed toward education, and another 25 percent are being directed toward the health sector (p. 10, IMF 2001). Social expenditures are expected to rise by almost twice the cash saving from the HIPC relief, suggesting that the countries are also putting fresh domestic resources into the socials sectors (p. 10, IMF

2001). Debt will be reduced by about two-thirds of the original debt stock (p. 6, IMF 2001). See IMF, "Heavily Indebted Poor Countries (HIPC) Initiative: Status of Implementation," May 25, 2001, available at http://www.imf.org/.

87. Thompson and Huber (2001), "Health Expenditure Trends in OECD Countries, 1970–1998," *HCFA Review*.

88. Lower-middle-income countries average $90 per person per year in health spending, and higher-middle-income countries average $240 per person per year. These sums are sufficient to ensure universal access to a core set of interventions.

89. There are other reasons as well. An excessive proportion of resources is directed at high-tech tertiary services, catering to urban elites, rather than to essential interventions needed by the poor. Also, there is simply a considerable amount of waste and misadministration as well.

90. Loans by the World Bank Group's non-concessional window (the International Bank for Reconstruction and Development) and by the regional development banks are made at the cost of the borrowed funds plus a small administrative fee. This is still at much lower interest rates and longer maturities than middle-income borrowers would get from private financial markets.

91. See Hanson, K., K Ranson, V. Oliveira, A, Mills, "Constraints to Scaling-Up Health Interventions: A Conceptual Framework and Empirical Analysis," CMH Working Paper Series No. WG5: 14, 2001, available at http://www.cid.harvard.edu

92. See D. Jamison and J. Wang, "Female Life Expectancy in a Panel of Countries, 1975-90," policy memorandum for the CMH (http://www.cid.harvard.edu). The authors find a striking effect of number of doctors per capita in extending life expectancy, as well as powerful geographical effects of tropics (adverse) and coastal proximity (favorable).

93. One important difference is that an island economy may be able to eliminate a disease vector while a mainland economy may suffer a continuing re-introduction of the vector over a land border with another country where the vector is not controlled.

94. Kerala, in the humid tropics, has such a surfeit of water resources that individuals have traditionally been able to bathe and rinse food extensively, and boil water in ample quantities. This may have helped Kerala to achieve its excellent health outcomes. In water-starved regions, these hygienic behaviors are likely to be much more expensive, and individuals may rely on the few available water holes, which may be pathogen-ridden as a result of the extensive human use.

95. On the other hand, the fact of globalization probably reduces the phenomenon of "virgin field" epidemics, in which a new pathogen is introduced into a population that has had no prior exposure, by an invading population with long-standing exposure to the disease. This often results in devastating effects on the "vir-

gin" population. Such was the case with European introductions of smallpox, measles, and other pathogens into the New World and Pacific Islands after 1500, where these introductions often led to the decimation of the indigenous populations.

96. The boundary between patentable and nonpatentable discoveries is currently subject to heated debate of great significance for future scientific inquiry. On the whole, we support a greater availability of basic, unpatented scientific knowledge to the whole world community.

97. There is a bipartisan consensus to double NIH annual funding between 1998 and 2003, from $13 billion in FY98 to $27 billion in FY03. The budget for fiscal year 2001 is $20.3 billion.

98. Many analysts have recently made the important distinction between diseases that are common to rich and poor countries—where rich-country R&D benefits the poor—and diseases that are basically exclusive to the poor countries, such as tropical parasitic diseases, where the level of R&D tends to be minimal. See Lanjouw (2001) for a useful analysis along these lines.

99. The ambiguity about malaria falling between Type II and Type III arises not from incidence, but from the fact that the rich-country market for prophylaxis and treatment for travelers and military personnel establishes a modest rich-country interest in malaria R&D.

100. DALYs, or disability-adjusted life years, associated with a disease are the number of life years lost because of premature mortality plus the number of life-year-equivalents lost due to chronic disability. Years lived with chronic disability are converted into an equivalent life years lost by a conversion factor reflecting the severity of the disability. As an example, a death of a male at age 30 is scored as 29.6 DALYs in the Global Burden of Disease study (1996, p. 17).

101. See Anderson, M. Maclean and C. Davies, 1996. *Malaria Research : An Audit of International Activity*. London: Wellcome Trust.

102. See Table 10 of this Report. A useful distinction here is between diseases that afflict both the high-income and low-income countries and diseases that afflict overwhelmingly the low-income countries. The first category of diseases will generally attract large-scale R&D within the rich countries themselves. The low-income countries can often "piggy back" on the technological advances developed for the high-income market, if they can afford to deploy the new technologies when they emerge. Examples of diseases that overlap rich and poor countries include measles, pneumococcal infections, and hepatitis B. Examples of disease of the poor include malaria and other tropical parasites. The second category of disease is the most neglected, since neither rich-country governments nor profit-oriented pharmaceutical companies have an incentive to invest in the necessary R&D.

103. A 90/10 split would suggest that as much as $6 billion per year is directed at diseases of the poor, but adding up the known amounts for malaria, tuberculosis, other tropical diseases, and other killer conditions in poor countries, it seems unlikely that the world total comes anywhere close to that sum. The estimate by the Commission on Health Research for Development was that, in 1986, $1.6 billion of $30 billion R&D worldwide was addressed to problems of the developing world. A similar study carried out at Harvard University in 1995 suggested that, in 1992, $2 billion of a worldwide $56 billion in health research was directed at the problems of the developing world. See Global Forum for Health Research 1999, pp. 46 and 69, for background and details.

104. TDR refers to the UNDP/World Bank/WHO Special Programme for Research and Training in Tropical Diseases. The eight targeted diseases are (with the share of budgeted expenditures for 1994–1997 in parentheses): malaria (50 percent), onchocerciasis (5 percent), Chagas disease (6 percent), schistosomiasis (10 percent), leprosy (4 percent), African trypanosomiasis (6 percent), filariasis (8 percent), and leishmaniasis (11 percent). Activities are guided by steering committees composed of leading independent international scientific experts. Recent accomplishments include the demonstrated effectiveness of the drug artemether against schistosome infections, and the evidence that combination drug therapy for malaria can produce significant gains in overall cure rates. For details, see http://www.who.int/tdr.

105. The WHO/UNAIDS Initiative for Vaccine Research (IVR) facilitates the development and introduction of vaccines against HIV, malaria, tuberculosis, pneumococcus, rotavirus, *Shigella* and other diarrheal agents, serotype A and B meningococcus, human papillomavirus, dengue, Japanese encephalitis, schistosomiasis, and leishmaniasis, and promotes the development of technologies to render immunization simpler and safer.

106. A recent study by the WHO-IFPMA (International Federation of Pharmaceutical Manufacturers Associations) Roundtable looked at the question of R&D priorities for diseases prevalent in poor countries. According to this study, priority areas for increased R&D include malaria, tuberculosis, lymphatic filariasis, onchocerciasis, leishmaniasis, schistosomiasis, African trypanosomiasis, Chagas' disease, nonspecific diarrheas, and GI nematode infestations. Malaria and tuberculosis have scientifically tractable targets for which substantially higher levels of R&D are justified. For African trypanosomiasis, Chagas disease, and leishmaniasis, current treatments are difficult to administer, have serious side effects, and are increasingly compromised by acquired resistance.

107. The US Orphan Drug Act (1983) defines "rare" disease as one that affects fewer than 200,000 people in the United States.

108. For a detailed discussion, see the Synthesis Paper of Working Group 2, and Kremer, M. Public Policies to Stimulate Development of Vaccines and Drugs for Neglected Diseases, CMH, July 2001.

109. World health increasingly requires global norms and standards, including International Health Regulations, the Codex Alimentarius (a WHO/FAO Commission on food safety), the Framework Convention on Tobacco Control, the WHO/UNICEF Code on Infant Feeding, and many other examples.

110. See the excellent brief overview of these issues in Roy Widdus, "Public-Private Partnerships for Health," *Bulletin of the World Health Organization,* Vol. 79, No. 8, 2001, 713–720.

111. See Amir Attaran and Lee Gillespie-White (2001, p. 286). Attaran and Gillespie-White find that only in South Africa are a large number of antiretroviral (ARV) patented (10 of 15 ARVs), mainly by Glaxo Wellcome, which patented products in a majority (up to 37 of 53 countries). Most ARVs in most countries are not under patent. Of the theoretical maximum of 795 patents (15 ARVs by 53 countries), only 172 patents were taken out, or 21.6 percent of the potential. For almost all countries, at least one standard triple combination could be obtained without patents covering any of the three drugs, and in most of the region several standard combinations would be available without patent protection. Still, some useful combinations are protected by patent, and this could certainly pose a complicating factor in scaling up treatment.

112. Activists have justly argued that drug pricing is an obstacle under any conditions of donor financing, since there are always some people in the low-income countries that are rationed out of access to essential medicines whenever prices are kept above the "lowest commercially viable price." Our point is that any large-scale access to the medicines by those that need them will require large-scale donor financing.

113. This is true even if cash-constrained donors rather than the low-income countries themselves are buying the drugs on behalf of the poor.

114. It may be argued that, since many new products are not currently patented in most low-income countries, the beginning of the enforcement of the TRIPS agreement will change little. We doubt this conclusion. Given the growing market in low-income countries that will come with increased donor support, pharmaceutical companies will become more likely take out patent protection as a matter of course, unless there are voluntary international understandings to the contrary.

115. Broad support for this conclusion was also expressed at the Workshop on Differential Pricing and Financing of Essential Drugs, organized by WHO and WTO, 8 to 11 April 2001, Hosbjor, Norway. As the Executive Summary of the Conference Report states, "there seemed to be a large amount of common thinking among participants on two central points: First, that differential pricing could, and should, play an important role in ensuring access to essential drugs at

affordable prices, especially in poor countries, while allowing the patent system to continue to play its role of providing incentives for research and development into new drugs; and Second, that while affordable prices are important, actually getting drugs, whether patented or generic, to the people who need them will require a major financing effort, both to buy the drugs and to reinforce health care supply systems, and that for these countries most of the additional financing will have to come from the international community." See http://www.who.int/ medicines/library/edm_general/who-wto-hosbjor/who-wto-hosbjor.html.

116. GlaxoSmithKline Plc granted a voluntary license to Aspen Pharmacare, South Africa's largest generic company, to produce GSK's antiretroviral drugs AZT and 3TC, and Combivir, which combines the two drugs into a single pill. "RPT-Glaxo gives up rights to AIDS drugs in South Africa," Ben Hirschler, Reuters, October 8, 2001.

117. See http://www.unaids.org/acc_access/index.html. The initial five companies involved in the Initiative were Boehringer Ingelheim, Bristol-Myers Squibb, GlaxoSmithKline, Merck & Co., and Hoffman-LaRoche.

118. International civil society, including groups such as CPTech and Health Gap (United States), *Médecins sans Frontières* and Oxfam (Europe), Treatment Access Campaign (South Africa), and Drug Study Group (Thailand), brought the urgency of the pricing issue to public attention, and contributed importantly to the recent progress on price reductions of essential medicines in low-income countries.

119. Several international partnerships for disease control have been organized around drug donation programs of pharmaceutical companies. These include: lymphatic filariasis (albendazole, GlaxoSmithKline); African trypanosomiasis (eflornithine, Aventis); leprosy (leprosy multidrug therapy, Novartis); malaria (atovaquone and proguanil, GlaxoSmithKline); onchocerciasis (ivermectin, Merck); Trachoma (azithromycin, Pfizer); mother-to-child transmission of HIV (nevaripine, Boehringer Ingelheim); fungal infections in HIV/AIDS patients (fluconazole, Pfizer). Other drug donations include oral polio vaccine (Aventis Pasteur), Hib vaccine (Wyeth Lederle Vaccines), and hepatitis B vaccine (Merck). There are also cases of other health products, for example autodestruct syringes for tetanus (Becton Dickenson) and nylon filter materials for guinea-worm prevention (Du Pont). In addition, there have been donations for training and infrastructure for HIV/AIDS (Merck and Bristol-Myers Squibb). See Initiative on Public-Private Partnerships for Health (IPPPH), info@ippph.org.

120. The *lowest viable commercial price* refers to the lowest price that makes it commercially viable to supply an incremental market on a sustained basis. This would generally equal the marginal cost of production plus handling expenses.

We would expect that middle-income countries would generally pay more than the low-income countries, but less than the rich countries. Prices in those markets would presumably be negotiated between suppliers and purchasers (e.g., government agencies), with the safeguard of compulsory licensing available for the middle-income countries. Such arrangements have recently led to the negotiation of significant price discounts for antiretrovirals in Brazil and some other middle-income countries compared with the prices in high-income countries.

121. A compulsory license does not require that the patent holder show the local producer how to produce the product. Thus the compulsory license is useful only if the product has been successfully "reverse engineered."

122. The UN Industrial Development Organization (UNIDO) has calculated that approximately one-third of the developing countries import 100 percent of the medicines they consume, and an additional one-third have very limited production capacity.

123. Assuming economic growth around 2.3 percent per year (2 percent per capita, 0.3 percent population) in the high-income countries, combined donor GNP should reach approximately $29 trillion in 2007, and $35 billion in 2015.

124. The single biggest recipient of World Bank AIDS financing during 1997–1999 was India, which received a $191 million concessional loan for the period 1999 to 2004.

125. "Transitional Arrangements" Report, meeting on the Global Fund to Fight AIDS, Tuberculosis, and Malaria (GFATM), Brussels, 12–13 July 2001.

126. Small amounts should go toward middle-income countries that for one reason or another (e.g., extraordinary incidence of disease or large pockets of recalcitrant poverty within the nation) are unable to cover their health needs out of national resources. For example, because of the AIDS pandemic, South Africa should be a recipient of funding for AIDS control.

127. http://www.vaccinealliance.org. GAVI is funded with approximately $1 billion, including $750 million from the Gates Foundation and $250 million from donor countries.

128. The Bank is now providing around $1.3 billion in new commitments per year in both IDA loans (concessional) and IBRD loans (nonconcessional) and currently has nearly $10 billion under commitment in health-sector projects. Ironically, IDA funds are actually underspent in many cases, signaling the reluctance of many impoverished countries to take on new debts (as opposed to grants) to finance expanded health coverage, as well as the need for a clearer multi-year framework for scaling up health services within which IDA financing would play a key, sustained and predictable role.

129. We note that the mere conversion of IDA loans to grants would not increase the Bank's net resource transfer to the low-income countries as a group (though it might make it easier for particular countries within the group of IDA-eligible countries). Currently, the Bank re-lends, at concessional rates, the amounts that it collects in debt repayments on IDA loans. It is easy to show that the net present value of resource transfers that the Bank makes through IDA are the same, whether they are made in one-time grants or in a sequence of concessional loans in which each new loan is made on the basis of repayments of the old loans. In either case, the present value of net resource transfers from IDA is just equal to the donor contributions to IDA in the first place, which backs the grants or loans. *The only way that IDA can make larger net resource transfers is for IDA's donors to contribute more funds to IDA in the first place, a policy that we support.*

130. Note that in this case we are talking about the production of health services domestically, not the importation of health services. Thus, even if total health outlays reach 12 percent of GNP, if half of the outlays are imported, then the value added originating in the health sector would be 6 percent of GNP.

131. The problem of brain drain is intense. In Ghana, for example, between 1998 and 2000, the number of medical doctors in the public sector declined from 1,400 to 1,115, and public-sector nurses from 17,000 to 12,600, with brain drain and transfer to the domestic private sector playing an important role. In general, public-sector wages of doctors and nurses in low-income countries are often less than one-third of the wages available in the domestic private sector, and perhaps one-tenth or less of the wages available in the international market if the doctor or nurse leaves the country for a job in a high-income economy.

132. The GNP of the low-income countries is currently around $1 trillion. If we suppose a population growth of 1 percent per annum and a per capita GNP growth of 2 percent per annum, the total GNP will grow by around 3 percent per annum. Twenty years of 3 percent growth per year would produce an aggregate GNP of $1.8 trillion.

133. Our experience in 2 years of work on the CMH has repeatedly demonstrated to us the value of placing the health issues within the context of the national budget as well as national social goals. Scaling up of health therefore requires the close collaboration of the Ministers of Health and Finance, as well as the collaboration of these ministries with leading groups in civil society. The consultation with civil society should include organizations representing those with the worst health problems, including women and marginalized ethnic or other groups. A National Commission on Macroeconomics and Health can provide an important venue for such coordinated work. Some countries may already have national committees on health that are part of the PRSP process, in which case these may cover the suggested functions of the NCMH, though we stress again the importance of both Ministers of Health and Finance participating jointly in the process.

Appendix 1: Participants, Reports, and Working Papers for the Commission on Macroeconomics and Health

Participants

Commissioners

Professor Jeffrey D. Sachs (Chair)
Galen L. Stone Professor of International Trade, Harvard University, and Director, Center for International Development at Harvard University, Cambridge, USA

Dr. Isher Judge Ahluwalia
Director, Indian Council for Research on International Economic Relations Indian Council for Research on International Economic Relations, New Delhi, India

Dr. K. Y. Amoako
Executive Secretary, United Nations Economic Commission for Africa United Nations Economic Commission for Africa, Addis Ababa, Ethiopia

Dr. Eduardo Aninat
(Former Minister of Finance, Chile)
Deputy Managing Director, International Monetary Fund
International Monetary Fund, Washington, DC, USA

Professor Daniel Cohen
Professor of Economics
Ecole normale supérieure, Paris, France

Mr. Zephirin Diabre
(Former Minister of Finance, Economy and Planning, Burkina Faso)
Associate Administrator, United Nations Development Program,
New York, USA

Dr. Eduardo Doryan
(Former Minister of Education, Costa Rica)
Special Representative of the World Bank to the United Nations
New York, USA

Professor Richard Feachem
(Former Dean, London School of Hygiene and Tropical Medicine)
Director, Institute of Global Health
University of California at San Francisco/University of California at Berkeley,
San Francisco, USA

Professor Robert W. Fogel
Professor of Economics, Center for Population Economics
University of Chicago, Chicago, USA

Professor Dean Jamison
Director, Center for Pacific Rim Studies
University of California, Los Angeles, USA

Mr. Takatoshi Kato
Senior Advisor, Bank of Tokyo-Mitsubishi Ltd.,
Tokyo, Japan

Dr. Nora Lustig
President, Universidad de las Américas-Puebla
Cholula, Mexico

Professor Anne Mills
Head, Health Economics and Financing Program
London School of Hygiene and Tropical Medicine, London, UK

Dr. Thorvald Moe

(Former Chief Economic Advisor and Deputy Permanent Secretary,
Norwegian Finance Ministry)
Deputy Secretary General, Organization for Economic Co-operation and
Development
Organization for Economic Co-operation and Development, Paris, France

Dr. Manmohan Singh

(Former Minister of Finance, India)
Member of Rajya Sabha
Government of India, New Delhi, India

Dr. Supachai Panitchpakdi

(Former Deputy Minister of Commerce, Thailand)
Director-General designate
World Trade Organization

Professor Laura Tyson

Dean, The Walter A. Haas School of Business
University of California at Berkeley, Berkeley, CA, USA

Dr. Harold Varmus

President, Memorial Sloan-Kettering Cancer Center, New York, USA

Chairman's team
Dr. Dyna Arhin-Tenkorang

Senior Economist CMH & Assistant to the Chairman of the CMH
Center for International Development at Harvard University, Boston, USA/
London School of Hygiene and Tropical Medicine, London, UK

Secretariat
Dr. Sergio Spinaci

Executive Secretary of the CMH
World Health Organization
Geneva, Switzerland

WG1 HEALTH, ECONOMIC GROWTH, AND POVERTY REDUCTION
This working group addressed the impact of health investments on poverty reduction and economic growth.

Co-Chairs
Sir George A. O. Alleyne, *Director, Pan American Health Organization, USA*
Professor Daniel Cohen, *Professor of Economics, Ecole normale supérieure, France*

Members
Dr. Dyna Arhin-Tenkorang, Senior Economist & Assistant to the Chairman of the CMH, Center for International Development at Harvard University, USA/ London School of Hygiene and Tropical Medicine, UK
Dr. Alok Bhargava, Department of Economics, University of Houston, USA
Dr. David E. Bloom, Professor of Economics and Demography, Department of Population and International Health, Harvard University, USA
Dr. David Canning, Professor of Economics, Queens University, Belfast, Northern Ireland
Dr. Juan A. Casas, Director of the Division of Health and Human Development, Pan American Health Organization, USA
Dr. Angus Deaton, Professor of Economics and Public Affairs, Princeton University, USA
Professor Dean T. Jamison, Director, Program on International Health and Education, University of California, USA
Dr. Gerald Keusch, Associate Director for International Research, National Institutes of Health; Director of the Fogarty International Center; Professor of Medicine, Tufts University of Medicine, USA
Dr. Felicia Knaul, Director, Center for Social and Economic Analysis of the Mexican Health Foundation, Mexico
Dr. Juan Luis Londoño, Engineer, Revista Dinero, Colombia
Dr. Nora Lustig, President, Universidad de las Américas-Puebla; formerly Senior Advisor and Chief, Poverty and Inequality, Unit of the Inter-American Development Bank (IABD), and Director, The World Development Report, The World Bank, USA

Dr. Mead Over, Senior Economist, Development Research Group, The
World Bank, USA

Professor Jeffrey D. Sachs, Professor of Economics and Director,
Center for International Development at Harvard University, USA

Dr. William Savedoff, Senior Economist, Financial Development
Division, Stop W0502, Inter-American Development Bank, USA

Professor Paul Schultz, Department of Economics, Yale University, USA

Professor Duncan Thomas, Department of Economics, University of
California, (UCLA), USA

Ms. Eva Wallstam, Director, Civil Society Initiative, World Health
Organization, Switzerland

WG2 GLOBAL PUBLIC GOODS FOR HEALTH

This working group studied "global public goods for health," that is,
multi-country policies, programs, and initiatives having a positive impact
on health that extends beyond the borders of any single country (e.g.,
international health research collaborations, smallpox eradication, etc).
Composed of sixteen members from academia, industry, nongovernmental organizations, and international agencies, the Working Group commissioned over twenty research papers in three major categories: research,
R&D for neglected products, and building research capacity in the developing countries; global aspects of communicable disease control and prevention; and information and dissemination of best practice.

Co-Chairs

Professor Richard Feachem, *Director, Institute for Global Health,*
University of California, USA

Professor Jeffrey D. Sachs, *Professor of Economics and Director, Center*
for International Development, Harvard University, USA

Program Director/Senior Researcher

Dr. Carol Medlin, *Institute for Global Health, University of California,*
USA

Members

Dr. Cristian Baeza, Regional Director, Latin America and the Caribbean
STEP Program, International Labor Organization, USA

Dr. John Barton, George E. Osbourne Professor of Law, Stanford Law
School, USA

Dr. Seth Berkley, President and CEO, International Aids Vaccine
Initiative, USA

Dr. Win Gutteridge, Area Coordinator: Product Research and
Development, Special Program for Research and Training in Tropical
Diseases, World Health Organization, Switzerland

Professor Dean T. Jamison, Director, Program on International Health
and Education, University of California, USA

Dr. Inge Kaul, Director, Office of Development Studies, United Nations
Development Program, USA

Dr. Gerald Keusch, Associate Director for International Research,
National Institutes of Health; Director of the Fogarty International
Center; Professor of Medicine, Tufts University of Medicine, USA

Dr. Ariel Pablo-Mendez, Associate Director, Health Equity, The
Rockefeller Foundation, USA

Dr. Geoffrey Lamb, Director, Finance and Resource Mobilization,
Department for International Development, The World Bank, UK

Dr. Adetokunbo O. Lucas, Adjunct Professor, Harvard University, USA

Dr. Bernard Pécoul, Director, Access to Essential Medicines, Médecins
sans Frontières

Dr. Sally Stansfield, Global Health Program Officer, Gates Foundation,
USA

Dr. David Webber, Director of Economic Policy and Fellow,
International Federation of Pharmaceutical Manufacturers
Association, Switzerland

Dr. Roy Widdus, Manager, Initiative on Public-Private Partnerships for
Health, Global Forum for Health Research, Switzerland

WG3 MOBILIZATION OF DOMESTIC RESOURCES FOR HEALTH

This Working Group assessed the economic consequences of alternative
approaches to resource mobilization for health systems and interventions
from domestic resources. This work was carried out in collaboration with
the International Monetary Fund and other institutions. It focused on how
health systems can best be financed at country level, including by reallo-
cation of public sector budgets and by expanding the role of the nongovernmental sector. Ongoing work in the Evidence and Information for
Policy (EIP) cluster of WHO provided an important input into this
Working Group.

Co-Chairs

Professor Kwesi Botchwey, *Director of Africa Research and Programs at Harvard Institute for International Development and the Center for International Development, USA*

Professor Alan Tait, *Honorary Professor at the University of Kent at Canterbury, and honorary Fellow of Trinity College, Dublin; Former Deputy Director of Fiscal Affairs, International Monetary Fund, Washington; and Former Director of IMF Office, Switzerland*

Members

Dr. Dyna Arhin-Tenkorang, Senior Economist & Assistant to the Chairman of the CMH, Center for International Development, Harvard University, USA

Professor Mukul Govindji Asher, Public Policy Program, National University of Singapore

Dr. Guido Carrin, Senior Health Economist, World Health Organization, Geneva, Switzerland

Mr. Sanjeev Gupta, Chief, Expenditure Policy Division, Fiscal Affairs Department, International Monetary Fund, USA

Mr. Peter S. Heller, Deputy Director, Fiscal Affairs Department, International Monetary Fund, USA

Professor William Hsiao, K.T. Li Professor of Economics, Department of Health Policy and Management, Harvard School of Public Health, USA

Ms. Rima Khalef Hunaidi, Assistant Secretary General / Director of the Regional Bureau for the Arab States, United Nations Development Programme, USA

Professor Dean T. Jamison, Director, Program on International Health and Education, University of California, USA

Dr. Juan Luis Londoño, Economist, Revista Dinero, Colombia

Mr. Rajiv Misra, Former Secretary, Ministry of Health, Gurgaon, India

Dr. Alexander S. Preker, Chief Economist, Health, Nutrition and Population, The World Bank, USA

Mr. George Schieber, Sector Manager, Health and Social Protection, The World Bank, USA

WG4 HEALTH AND THE INTERNATIONAL ECONOMY
This group examined trade in health services, health commodities and
health insurance; patents for medicines and Trade-Related Intellectual
Property Rights (TRIPS); international movements of risk factors; international migration of health workers; health conditions and health finance
policies as rationales for protection; and other ways that trade may be
impacting on the health sector. Ongoing work at WHO and WTO provided important inputs into this Working Group.

Chair
Dr. Isher Judge Ahluwalia, *Director and Chief Executive, Indian Council*
for Research on International Economic Relations, India

Members
Dr. Harvey Bale, Director-General, International Federation of
  Pharmaceutical Manufacturers' Association, Switzerland
Dr. John Barton, Professor of Law, Stanford Law School, USA
Dr. Tony Culyer, Professor of Economics, University of York,
  University of Toronto, Canada
Ms. Ellen 't Hoen, LL.M., Access to Essential Medicines Campaign,
  Médecins sans Frontières
Dr. Calestous Juma, Director, Science and Technology and Innovation
  Program, Center for International Development, Harvard University;
  Research Fellow, Belfast Center for Science and International Affairs,
  Harvard University, USA
Dr. Keith E. Maskus, Lead Economist, DECRG, The World Bank,
  Washington DC, USA
Dr. Supachai Panitchpakdi, World Trade Organization Director-General
  Designate, former Deputy Prime Minister and Minister of Commerce,
  Thailand
Dr. Arvind Panagariya, Professor and Co-Director, Center for
  International Economics, Department of Economics, University of
  Maryland, USA
Dr. John Sbarbaro, Professor of Medicine and Preventive Medicine,
  University of Colorado, USA
Dr. Jacques van der Gaag, Professor of Development Economics, Dean
  of the Faculty of Economics and Econometrics, University of
  Amsterdam, The Netherlands

Dr. Richard Wilder, Director, Powell, Goldstein, Frazer and Murphy, Washington, USA

Mr. B. K. Zutshi, Former Ambassador and PR of India to GATT, and Advisor, Indian Council for Research on International Economic Relations, India

WG5 IMPROVING HEALTH OUTCOMES OF THE POOR
This group examined the technical options, constraints, and costs for mounting a major global effort to improve the health of the poor dramatically by 2015. It undertook analyses of avoidable mortality, identified available interventions to address the key causes, reviewed evidence on how to relax constraints, and estimated the costs of scaling up coverage of key interventions along with the costs of the required system strengthening. It drew extensively on ongoing work within WHO, at the World Bank, and within international schools of public health.

Co-Chairs

Professor Anne Mills, *Head of Health Economics and Financing Programme, London School of Hygiene and Tropical Medicine, UK, and CMH member*

Dr. Prabat Jha, *Senior Scientist, World Health Organization, Switzerland*

Members

Dr. Mushtaque Chowdhury, Deputy Executive Director and Director of Research, BRAC, Bangladesh

Dr. Jorge Jimenez de la Jara, Professor, Department of Public Health, Catholic University of Chile, Chile

Dr. Peter Kilima, Regional Co-ordinator for Anglophone Africa, International Trachoma Initiative, Tanzania

Dr. Jeffrey Koplan, Director, Centers for Disease Control, USA

Dr. Ayanda Ntsaluba, Director-General of Health Services, National Department of Health, South Africa

Mr. Ram Ramasundaram, Joint Secretary, Department of Commerce, India

Dr. Sally Stansfield, Senior Program Officer, Bill and Melinda Gates Foundation, USA

Dr. Jaime Galvez Tan, Professor, University of the Philippines College of Medicine, and President, Health Futures Foundation Inc., Philippines

Professor Marcel Tanner, Director, Swiss Tropical Institute, Switzerland

WG6 DEVELOPMENT ASSISTANCE AND HEALTH
This group reviewed health implications of development assistance policies including modalities relating to debt relief. It focused on the policies
and approaches of international developmental agencies. One emphasis
was on the appropriate balance between country-specific work and support for activities that address international provision of global public
goods. The Working Group drew on ongoing work within WHO, the
World Bank, international schools of public health, and research units of
aid agencies.

Co-Chairs
Mr. Zephirin Diabre, *Associate Administrator, United Nations
Development Program, USA*
Mr. Christopher Lovelace, *Director, Health, Nutrition and Population,
The World Bank, USA*
Ms. Carin Norberg, *Director, Democracy and Social Development,
Swedish International Development Agency, Stockholm, Sweden*

Members
Dr. Dyna Arhin-Tenkorang, Senior Economist & Assistant to the
Chairman of the CMH, Center for International Development at
Harvard University, USA / London School of Hygiene and Tropical
Medicine, UK
Dr. Ingar Bruggerman, Director, International Planned Parenthood
Federation, UK
Dr. Andrew Cassels, Director, Sustainable Development & Healthy
Environments, World Health Organization, Switzerland
Dr. Nick Drager, Department of Health and Development, World Health
Organization, Switzerland
Mr. Björn Ekman, Economist, Department for Democracy and Social
Development, Swedish International Development Cooperation
Agency, Sweden
Dr. Tim Evans, Director, Health Sciences, Rockefeller Foundation, USA
Mr. Paul Isenman, Head, Strategic Management of Development Co-
operation Division, Development Cooperation Directorate, OECD,
France
Dr. Inge Kaul, Director, Office of Development Studies, United Nations
Development Programme, USA

Dr. Julian Lob-Levyt, Chief Health and Population Advisor, Department for International Development, UK

Dr. Anders Nordstrom, Swedish International Development Cooperation Agency, Sweden

Mr. Ingvar Theo Olsen, Norwegian Agency for Development Cooperation, Norway

Dr. Susan Stout, Lead Implementation Specialist, World Bank, USA

Dr. H. Sudarshan, Director, VGKK (a health trust for indigenous people in Karnataka), India

Dr. A. Issaka-Tinorgah, Former Ag. Director of Medical Services, Ministry of Health, Ghana

Ms. Eva Wallstam, Director, Civil Society Initiative, World Health Organization, Switzerland

Biographical Sketches

Isher Judge Ahluwalia

Isher Judge Ahluwalia is Director and Chief Executive, Indian Council for Research on International Economic Relations (ICRIER), New Delhi. A graduate of the Delhi School of Economics and the Massachusetts Institute of Technology, Dr. Ahluwalia has spent the last 15 years writing books as well as articles in professional journals on the Indian economy. Her book, *Industrial Growth in India: Stagnation Since the Mid-Sixties* (Oxford University Press, 1985), received the Batheja Memorial Award for the best book on the Indian economy in 1987. Recently, Dr. Ahluwalia co-edited the volume *India's Economic Reforms and Development: Essays for Manmohan Singh* (Oxford University Press, 1998) with Prof. I.M.D. Little of Oxford University.

Dr. Ahluwalia has held several important nonexecutive positions on the boards of governors of public sector enterprises, research institutions, and financial institutions. Among her important assignments at present are Non Executive Director on the Board of Steel Authority of India Ltd. (SAIL); Member, Governing Body, National Institute of Public Finance & Policy (NIPFP); and Member, Governing Body, Institute of Economic Growth. Dr. Ahluwalia is a member of the Planning Board of Punjab and of the Advisory Committees to the Chief Ministers of Andhra Pradesh, Rajasthan, and Chattisgarh.

K. Y. Amoako

Since 1995, K. Y. Amoako has been Executive Secretary of the Economic Commission for Africa (ECA), the regional arm of the United Nations in Africa, at the rank of Under-Secretary-General of the United Nations. Prior to his work with the ECA, he served in the World Bank for several years, most recently in senior positions including Director of the Education and Social Policy Department with responsibility for providing strategic leadership for the Bank's programs on poverty reduction and human resource development (1993–1995); Division Chief of the Human Resources Operations Division for Brazil, Venezuela and Peru (1990–1992); and Division Chief for Country Operations for six countries in eastern Africa (1985–1990). K.Y. Amoako received his B.A. (Hons) with a concentration in Economics from the University of Ghana in Legon, and his M.A. and Ph.D. degrees in Economics from the University of California at Berkeley.

Eduardo Aninat

Eduardo Aninat is the Deputy Managing Director of the International Monetary Fund (IMF). Dr. Aninat was previously the Finance Minister of Chile. He served as the Chairman of the Board of Governors of the IMF and the World Bank in 1995–1996 and, for 3 years, as a member of the Development Committee of the World Bank and the IMF, representing Chile, Argentina, Bolivia, Peru, Uruguay, and Paraguay. Dr. Aninat previously served in a range of economic positions in the Chilean Government, including Chief Senior Negotiator for the bilateral Canada-Chile trade agreement, and Chief Debt Negotiator and Senior Advisor of the Central Bank of Chile and the Ministry of Finance. He has acted as a consultant for such international institutions as the World Bank and the Inter-American Development Bank, and as an advisor to a number of governments on matters ranging from tax policy to debt restructuring. He was also a member of the Board of Directors of the Institute of the Americas and a contributing editor to its official magazine. Dr. Aninat currently serves as the President of the Social Equity Forum (SEF). He has taught Public Finance and Economic Development at the Pontificia Universidad Católica de Chile and was an Assistant Professor of Economics at Boston University. He has an M.A. and Ph.D. in Economics from Harvard University.

Daniel Cohen

Daniel Cohen is Professor of Economics, Université de Paris (Panthéon-Sorbonne) and Ecole normale supérieure, Paris. He is also a member of the Council of Economic Analysis of the French Prime Minister, and an op-ed columnist to Le Monde magazine. Professor Cohen was a distinguished fellow of the Association Française de Sciences Economiques in 1987, and was appointed "Economist of the Year" in 1997 by Le Nouvel Economiste. From 1991 to 1998, he was the co-director of the International Macroeconomics Programme at the Center for Economic Policy Research (CEPR). Professor Cohen also served as a consultant to the World Bank from 1984 to 1997. He has served as an advisor to the Bolivian Government (along with Jeffrey D. Sachs), and was a Visiting

Scholar at Harvard University from 1981 to 1982. He has published several books, including *Private Lending to Sovereign States*, *Our Modern Times*, and *The Wealth of the World and the Poverty of Nations*, the last of which has been translated into 15 languages.

Zephirin Diabre

Zephirin Diabre, a national from Burkina Faso, has been the United Nations Development Programme (UNDP) Associate Administrator since 1999. Prior to entering the UN, he held several senior public posts in his country, serving as Advisor to the President of Burkina Faso (1998); President of the national Economic and Social Council (1996–1997); Minister of the Economy, Finance and Planning (1994–1996); and Minister of Trade, Industry and Mines (1992–1994). Founder of the Burkina Management Association and of the Burkina/France Business Association, Mr. Diabre also has experience in the private sector as Director for Human Resources of the Burkina Brewery Corporation. Mr. Diabre was a Visiting Scholar at the Harvard Institute for International Development and a Fellow of the Weatherhead Center for International Affairs in 1997.

Eduardo A. Doryan

Eduardo A. Doryan is Special Representative of the World Bank to the United Nations in New York, and was Vice President of the World Bank, formerly heading the Human Development Network (health, nutrition, population, education and social protection). Previously he served as the Deputy Minister for Science and Technology, and, years later, as Minister for Education in Costa Rica. He has been a professor both at the University of Costa Rica and at the Central American Institute for Business Administration (INCAE). He has a Ph.D. in Political Economy and Government from Harvard University.

Richard G. A. Feachem

Richard G. A. Feachem is the founding Director of the Institute for Global Health, a joint initiative of the University of California, San Francisco and the University of California, Berkeley. He is also Professor of International Health at UCSF and UC Berkeley. Previously, Dr. Feachem was Director of Health, Nutrition and Population at the World Bank (1995–1999) and Dean of the London School of Hygiene and Tropical Medicine (1989–1995). Dr. Feachem has also worked at the Universities of New

South Wales and Birmingham and the World Health Organization. Dr. Feachem has served on many boards and committees. He currently serves on the Council of Voluntary Service Overseas, the Health Advisory Committee of the British Council, the Board of the International AIDS Vaccine Initiative, and the Board on Global Health of the US Institute of Medicine. He is also the Chair of the Advisory Board of the Initiative on Public Private Partnerships for Health, and Chair of the Foundation Council of the Global Forum for Health Research. Since 1999, Professor Feachem has been Editor-in-Chief of the *Bulletin of the World Health Organization*. Professor Feachem's interests are in international health and development. He has published extensively in these and other fields. He holds the following degrees: CBE, FREng, BSc, PhD, DSc (Med), FICE, FIWEM, and Hon FFPHM.

Robert William Fogel
Robert William Fogel received his B.A. from Cornell University, his M.A. from Columbia University, and his Ph.D., in Economics, from Johns Hopkins University. He has held faculty positions at the University of Rochester, Cambridge University, and Harvard University. He is currently the Charles R. Walgreen Distinguished Service Professor of American Institutions in the Graduate School of Business, Director of the Center for Population Economics, and a member of the Department of Economics and of the Committee on Social Thought at the University of Chicago. He is also co-director of the Program on Cohort Studies at the National Bureau of Economic Research. He received the Nobel Prize in Economics in 1993 (with Douglas C. North). During his graduate work under Simon Kuznets, he became interested in combining the study of economics and history to understand long-term technological and institutional change. Since the late 1980s, his principal research has focused on explaining the secular decline in mortality and the changing pattern of aging over the life cycle in the United States. The latest findings from this project are scheduled to be published in 2002 in a book entitled *The Escape from Hunger and Premature Death 1700-2100: Europe, America, and the Third World*. His other current research includes a study of the high-performing Asian economies, research into nutrition and longevity, and historical work on the development of the discipline of economics in the 20th century.

Dean T. Jamison

Dean T. Jamison has been a Professor at the University of California, Los Angeles, since 1988. He directs UCLA's Program on Global Health and Education, and teaches both International Health Economics and Economics of Education. Earlier in his career, Jamison spent many years at the World Bank where he was a Senior Economist in the Research Department, Health Project Officer for China and for Gambia, Division Chief for Education Policy, and Division Chief for Population, Health and Nutrition. In 1992—1993, he temporarily rejoined the World Bank to serve as lead author for the Bank's 1993 World Development Report, *Investing in Health*. During 1998–2000, Jamison was on partial leave from UCLA to serve as Director, Economics Advisory Service at the World Health Organization in Geneva. At present, in addition to his UCLA position, Jamison is a Fellow of the Bill and Melinda Gates Foundation and a Senior Fellow at the Fogarty International Center of the US National Institutes of Health. Jamison studied at Stanford (A.B. in Philosophy; M.S. in Engineering Sciences) and at Harvard (Ph.D. in Economics, under Nobel laureate K. J. Arrow). In 1994, he was elected to membership in the Institute of Medicine of the US National Academy of Sciences.

Takatoshi Kato

Mr. Takatoshi Kato is currently Adviser to the President, the Bank of Tokyo-Mitsubishi and also Visiting Professor in Asia-Pacific Studies, Waseda University. He was also Weinberg Visiting Professor, Woodrow Wilson School, Princeton University for the 1998/1999 school year.

Mr. Kato was Japan's G7 Deputy in 1995–1997 as Vice Minister of Finance for International Affairs. In his 34 years of Japanese Government service, he assumed numerous positions, including Director-General, International Finance Bureau (1993–1995) and Executive Director at the Asian Development Bank (1985–1987). Mr. Kato received his L.L.B. from Tokyo University and his M.P.A. from Woodrow Wilson School, Princeton University.

Nora Lustig

Nora Lustig is the President of the Universidad de las Américas-Puebla, Mexico. Previously Dr. Lustig was the Senior Advisor and Chief of the Poverty and Inequality Unit at the Inter-American Development Bank. She was a Senior Fellow in the Foreign Policy Studies Program at the Brookings Institution and was Professor of Economics at El Colegio de

Mexico in Mexico City. She was also a Visiting Research Scholar at the Massachusetts Institute of Technology in 1982 and a Visiting Professor at the University of California, Berkeley, in 1984.

Nora Lustig was co-director of the World Bank's World Development Report 2000/2001 *"Attacking Poverty."* She was also co-founder and President of the Latin American and Caribbean Economic Association (LACEA) between 1998 and 1999, and is currently co-director of the LACEA Network on Inequality, Poverty and Economic Mobility. She is a non-Resident Senior Fellow in the Foreign Policy Studies Program at the Brookings Institution and a Senior Associated Fellow of the Inter-American Dialogue. Dr. Lustig is a member of the Board of the World Institute on Development Economics Research (WIDER), of the Commission on Macroeconomics and Health at the World Health Organization, and of the Group of Experts at the International Labor Office.

Dr. Lustig has published extensively on development economics, with a particular focus on Latin America. Her book entitled *Mexico: The Remaking of an Economy* received *Choice Magazine's* 1994 Outstanding Book Award. Born in Buenos Aires, Argentina, Dr. Lustig has also lived in Mexico and the United States. She received her Ph.D. in Economics from the University of California, Berkeley.

Anne Mills

Anne Mills is Professor of Health Economics and Policy at the London School of Hygiene and Tropical Medicine, and Head of the Health Economics and Financing Programme, which together with its many research partners, has a large program of research focused on equity and efficiency of health systems in low and middle income countries. She has nearly 30 years of experience in health-economics related research in low- and middle-income countries, and has published widely in the fields of health economics and policy. Her current research interests are in the organization and financing of health systems and the economic analysis of disease control activities, especially for malaria. She has had extensive involvement in supporting capacity development in health economics in low- and middle-income countries, and has acted as advisor to many multilateral and bilateral agencies.

Thorvald Moe

Thorvald Moe is one of the four Deputy Secretaries-General of the Organisation for Economic Co-operation and Development (OECD) based in Paris. Within OECD, he is, among other things, responsible for overseeing work on education, employment, and the environment, and for a major program of work on sustainable development in which most OECD Directorates are working closely together. Before taking his current appointment in 1998, Dr. Moe had been Chief Economic Adviser and Deputy Permanent Secretary at the Norwegian Finance Ministry since 1989. From 1986 to 1989, he was Norway's Ambassador to the OECD. From 1973 to 1986, Dr. Moe served in the Finance Ministry as Deputy, and then Director General, for the Economic Policy Department following a period in the Budget Department. Dr. Moe has written and contributed to several books and many papers and articles on topics including macro-economic policies, employment policies, the effects of demographics on economic growth to public planning and budgeting, the economics of climate change, and the relationship between environmental policies and employment. He has been on numerous boards, commissions, and committees in Norway and internationally, including the Economic Policy Committee of the OECD. Dr. Moe holds a B.A. in Economics from the University of California at Los Angeles and a Ph.D. in Economics from Stanford University.

Jeffrey D. Sachs

Jeffrey D. Sachs is the Director of the Center for International Development at Harvard University, the Galen L. Stone Professor of International Trade at Harvard University, former Director of the Harvard Institute for International Development, and a Research Associate of the National Bureau of Economic Research. Dr. Sachs serves as an economic advisor to several governments in Latin America, eastern Europe, the Former Soviet Union, Africa, and Asia. He was cited in *The New York Times Magazine* as "probably the most important economist in the world" and in a *Time Magazine* issue on 50 promising young leaders as "the world's best-known economist." Sachs is the recipient of many awards and honors, including membership in the Harvard Society of Fellows, the American Academy of Arts and Sciences, and the Fellows of the World Econometric Society. He received Honorary Degrees from St. Gallen University in Switzerland, Lingnan College in Hong Kong, Iona College in New York, and Varna Economic University in Bulgaria. In September 1991, he was honored with the Frank E. Seidman Award in Political Economy. He has delivered the prestigious Lionel Robbins Memorial Lectures at the London School of Economics, the John Hicks

Lectures at Oxford University, the David Horowitz Lectures in Tel Aviv, the Frank D. Graham Lectures at Princeton University, and the Tanner Lectures at the University of Utah. Dr. Sachs received his B.A., *summa cum laude*, from Harvard College in 1976, and his M.A. and Ph.D. from Harvard University in 1978 and 1980, respectively. He joined the Harvard faculty as an Assistant Professor in 1980, and was promoted to Associate Professor in 1982 and Full Professor in 1983. He is currently Chair of the Commission on Macroeconomics and Health of the World Health Organization for the years 2000–2001, and from September 1999 through March 2000, he served as a member of the International Financial Institutions Advisory Commission established by the US Congress.

Manmohan Singh

Manmohan Singh is currently the Leader of Opposition, Rajya Sabha (Council of States) Parliament of India. He has previously served in many other positions of the Indian Government, including Finance Minister, Advisor to the Prime Minister of India on Economic Affairs, Secretary, Ministry of Finance and Governor of the Reserve Bank of India, Deputy Chairman of Indian Planning Commission, and Chief Economic Adviser to India's Ministry of Finance. Dr. Singh has also received a number of awards, including the Justice K. S. Hegde Foundation Award, the Nikkei Asia Prize for Regional Growth, and the Jawaharlal Nehru Birth Centenary Award of the Indian Science Congress Association. He garnered the 1993 Euromoney Award for Finance Minister of the Year, and twice received the Asiamoney Award for Finance Minister of the Year (1993, 1994). Dr. Singh has been presented with a number of honorary degrees from institutions all over the world. He holds a B.A. and M.A. in Economics from Punjab and Cambridge Universities and a D.Phil from the University of Oxford.

H. E. Supachai Panitchpakdi

Supachai Panitchpakdi is currently the Director-General Designate of the World Trade Organization. Dr. Supachai Panitchpakdi was formerly the Deputy Prime-Minister and Minister of Commerce for Thailand. He has also held various positions in the private sector, such as the President of the Thai Military Bank, Chairman of Nava Finance and Securities, and Chairman of the Commercial Union. Dr. Supachai Panitchpakdi received his Master's Degree and Ph.D. in Econometrics and Development Planning from Erasmus University in Rotterdam, The Netherlands. In

1973, he was a Visiting Fellow to the Department of Econometrics at Cambridge University.

Laura Tyson

Dr. Laura Tyson is the current Dean of the Walter A. Haas School of Business at the University of California, Berkeley, and, in December 2001, will become Dean of the London School of Business. Tyson joined the UC Berkeley faculty in 1977 and currently holds the Class of 1939 Chair in Economics and Business Administration. She took leave from UC Berkeley in 1993, when President Clinton appointed her chairman of the White House Council of Economic Advisors. She was the first woman to hold that post. In 1995, Tyson succeeded Robert Rubin as National Economic Advisor. In accepting that position, Tyson became the highest-ranking woman in the Clinton White House. Tyson is the author of *Who's Bashing Whom? Trade Conflicts in High-Technology Industries* (Institute for International Economics, 1992) and numerous other works on economic competitiveness. Tyson recently was named one of four White House appointees to the National Bipartisan Commission on the Future of Medicare. She is a principal of the Law & Economics Consulting Group and a member of the boards of directors of Ameritech Corporation, the Council on Foreign Relations, Eastman Kodak Company, the Institute for International Economics, the John D. and Catherine T. MacArthur Foundation, and Morgan Stanley, Dean Witter, Discover & Co. Before her appointments in Washington DC, Tyson served at UC Berkeley as Research Director of the Berkeley Roundtable on the International Economy (BRIE) and as Director of the Institute of International Studies. Tyson received her B.A. in Economics, *summa cum laude*, in 1969 from Smith College in Massachusetts and her Ph.D. in Economics in 1974 from the Massachusetts Institute of Technology.

Harold Varmus

Harold Varmus has served as the President and Chief Executive Officer of Memorial Sloan-Kettering Cancer Center in New York City since January 2000. A former Director of the National Institutes of Health (NIH), in 1989 Dr. Varmus received the Nobel Prize for Physiology or Medicine, sharing the award with co-recipient Dr. J. Michael Bishop for their work on the genetic basis of cancer. In 1993, Varmus was named by President Clinton to serve as the Director of the National Institutes of Health, a position he held until the end of 1999. In addition to writing over 300 scientific papers and four books, including an introduction to the genetic basis of cancer for a general audience, Varmus has been an advisor to the Federal government, pharmaceutical and biotechnology firms, and many academic institutions. He has been a member of the US National Academy of Sciences since 1984 and of the Institute of Medicine since 1991. Dr. Varmus earned a B.A. in English from Amherst College and an M.A. in English from Harvard University. He is a graduate of Columbia University's College of Physicians and Surgeons and served on the medical house staff at Columbia-Presbyterian Hospital. His scientific training occurred first as a Public Health Service Officer at the NIH, where he studied bacterial gene expression with Dr. Ira Pastan, and then as a postdoctoral fellow with Dr. Bishop at the University of California, San Francisco.

Reports and Working Papers

Working Paper Series
Papers submitted and available at www.cid.harvard.edu and at
www.cmhealth.org.

Paper 8: Health, Human Capital, and Economic Growth (**Bloom DE, Canning D**)

Paper 9: Health, Longevity and Life-Cycle Savings (**Bloom DE, Canning D**)

Paper 10: The Economic Burden of Malaria (**Gallup, JL, Sachs, JD**)

Paper 11: The Effects of Early Nutritional Intervention on Human Capital Formation Institute of Nutrition of Central America and Panama (**INCAP**)

Paper 12: Responding to the Burden of Mental Illness (**Whiteford H, Teeson M, Scheurer R, Jamison D**)

Paper 13: The Effect of the AIDS Epidemic on Economic Welfare in Sub-Saharan Africa (**Wang J**)

Paper 14: Nutrition, Health, and Economic Development: Some Policy Priorities (**Bhargava A**)

Paper 15: AIDS and Economics (**Bloom DE, Mahal A, Sevilla J, River Path Associates**)

Working Group 2

Paper 1: A Conceptual Framework for Understanding Global and Transnational Goods for Health (**Sandler T, Arce D**)

Paper 2: International Collaboration in Health Research (**Lucas AO**)

Paper 3: Scientific Capacity Building to Improve Population Health: Knowledge as a Global Public Good (**Freeman P, Miller M**)

Paper 4: Ethics in International Health Research: A Perspective from the Developing World (**Bhutta ZA**)

Paper 5: Cultures of Ethical Conduct in Research: A Proposal for Progress in International Collaborative Research (**Lavery JV**)

Paper 6: The Role of Intellectual Property and Licensing in Promoting Research in International Health: Perspectives from a Public Sector Biomedical Research Agency (**Keusch GT, Nugent RA**)

Paper 7: Public Policies to Stimulate the Development of Vaccines and Drugs for the Neglected Diseases (**Kremer M**)

Paper 8: Orphan Drug Laws in Europe and the US: Incentives for the Research and Development of Medicines for the Diseases of Poverty (**Milne C, Kaiten K, Ronchi E**)

Paper 9: Differential Pricing for Pharmaceuticals: Reconciling Access, R&D, and Intellectual Property (**Danzon P**)

Paper 10: A Patent Proposal for Global Diseases (**Lanjouw JO**)

Paper 11: TRIPS and R&D Incentives in the Pharmaceutical Sector
(**Correa C**)

Paper 12: Patents in Genomics and Basic Research: Issues for Global
Health (**Barton J**)

Paper 13: International Scientific Cooperation: Considerations from
Previous Efforts (**Barton J, Heumueller D**)

Paper 14: The Epidemiological Basis of Communicable Disease Control
in Relation to Global Public Goods for Health (**Bradley D**)

Paper 15: International Coordination to Control Communicable Disease
(**St. John R, Plant A**)

Paper 16: Global Responses to the Growing Threat of Antimicrobial
Resistance (**Smith RD, Coast J**)

Paper 17: International Law and Global Infectious Disease Control
(**Fidler D**)

Paper 18: Global Information Needs for Health (**Musgrove P**)

Paper 19: The Evolving Role of the International Agencies in Supplying
and Financing Global Public Goods for Health (**Bumgarner R**)

Paper 20: Public-Private Partnership to Promote R&D Activity
(**Kettler H, Towse A**)

Paper 21: Innovative Financing of Global Public Goods for Health
(**Stansfield S, Harper M, Lamb G, Lob-Levyt J**)

Working Group 3

Paper 1: Mobilizing Resources for Health: The Case for User Fees Re-
visited (**Arhin-Tenkorang DC**)

Paper 2: Health Insurance for the Informal Sector in Africa: Design
Features, Risk Protection and Resource Mobilization (**Arhin-
Tenkorang DC**)

Paper 3: The Debt Relief Initiative and Public Health Spending in
Heavily Indebted Poor Countries (HIPCs) (**Gupta S, Clements B,
Guin-Siu MT, Leruth L**)

Paper 4: The Impact of the Degree of Risk-Sharing in Health Financing
on Health System Attainment (**Carrin G, Zeramdini R, Musgrove P,
Poullier J-P, Valentine N, Xu, K**)

Paper 5: Financing Health Systems through Efficiency Gains
(**Hensher M**)

Paper 6: Unmet Health Needs of Two billion: Is Community Financing a
Solution? (**Hsiao WC**)

Paper 7: A Strategic Framework in Mobilizing Domestic Resources for Health (**Hsiao WC**)

Paper 8 : Strategic Issues in Financing Health in Middle and High Income Countries (**Jamison D**)

Paper 9: Community Involvement in Health Care Financing: Impact, Strengths and Weaknesses: A Survey of the Literature (**Jakab M, Krishnan C**)

Paper 10: Social Inclusion and Financial Protection Through Community Financing: Initial Results from Five Household Surveys (**Jakab M, Preker, AS, Krishnan C, Schneider P, Diop F, Jutting J, Gumber A, Ranson K, Supakankunti S**)

Paper 11: A Summary Description of Health Financing in WHO Member States (**Musgrove P, Zeramdini R**)

Paper 12: A Synthesis Report on the Role of Community in Resource Mobilization and Risk Sharing (**Preker AS, Carrrin G, Dror D, Jakab M, Hsiao W, Arhin-Tenkorang D**)

Paper 13: The Global Expenditure Gap in Securing Financial Protection and Access to Health Care for the Poor (**Preker AS, Langenbrunner J, Suzuki E**)

Paper 14: Mobilisation of Domestic Resources for Health through Taxation: A Summary Survey (**Tait AA**)

Working Group 4

Paper 1: Post-TRIPS Options for Access to Patented Medicines in Developing Countries (**Scherer FM, Watal J**)

Paper 2: Differentiated Pricing of Patented Products (**Barton JH**)

Paper 3: Consumption and Trade in Off-Patented Medicines (**Bale H**)

Paper 4: Protection of Traditional Medicine (**Wilder R**)

Paper 5: Trade in Health Services (**Chanda R**)

Paper 6: Globalization and Health: A Survey of Opportunities and Risks for the Poor in Developing Countries (**Diaz-Bonilla E, Babinard J, Pinstrup-Andersen P**)

Paper 7: Trade Liberalization in Health Insurance: Opportunities and Challenges in Middle and Low Income Countries (**Sbarbaro J**)

Paper 8: The Role of Information Technology in Designs of Healthcare Trade (**Mathur A**) (under preparation)

Background Note 1: Trade Barriers and Prices of Essential Health Sector Inputs (**Woodward D**)

Background Note 2: Globalization and Health: A Framework for Analysis and Action (**Woodward D, Drager N, Beaglehole R, Lipson DJ**)

Background Note 3: Confronting the Tobacco Epidemic in an Era of Trade Liberalization (**Bettcher D, Subramanian C, Guindon E, Perucic A-M, Soll L, Grabman G, Joossens L, Taylor A**)

Background Note 4: GATS and Trade in Health Insurance Services (**Lipson DJ**)

Working Group 5

Paper 1: Avoidable Mortality in India (**Jha P, Nguyen S**)

Paper 2: The Evidence Base for Interventions to Prevent HIV Infection in Low and Middle Income Countries (**Jha P, Vaz LME, Plummer F, Nagelkerke N, Willbond B, Ngugi E, Prasado Rao JVR, Moses S, John G, Nduati R, MacDonald KS, Berkley S**)

Paper 3: The Evidence Base of Interventions for Care and Management of AIDS in Low and Middle Income Countries (**Willbond B, Plummer FA**)

Paper 4: Modelling the HIV/AIDS Epidemics in India and Botswana: The Effect of Interventions (**Nagelkerke N, Jha P, de Vlas S, Korenromp E, Moses S, Blanchard J, Plummer F**)

Paper 5: Maternal and Neonatal Mortality in Low and Middle Income Countries (**Gelband H**)

Paper 6: The Evidence Base for Interventions to Reduce Malaria Mortality in Low and Middle Income Countries (**Meek S, Hill J, Webster J**)

Paper 7: The Evidence Base for Interventions to Reduce Smoking-Related Mortality in Low and Middle Income Countries (**Chaloupka FJ, Jha P, Corrao MA, Costa e Silva V, Ross H, Czart C, Yach D**)

Paper 8: The Evidence Base for Interventions to Reduce Tuberculosis Mortality in Low and Middle Income Countries: Effectiveness, Cost-Effectiveness, and Constraints to Scaling Up (**Borgdorff MW, Floyd K, Broekmans JF**)

Paper 9: The Evidence Base for Interventions to Reduce Under Five Mortality in Low and Middle Income Countries (**Gelband H, Stansfield S, Nemer L, Jha P**)

Paper 10: The Evidence Base for Interventions to Mortality from Vaccine-Preventable Diseases in Low and Middle Income Countries (**England S, Loevinsohn B, Melgaard B, Kou U, Jha P**)

Paper 11: The Evidence Base for Interventions to Reduce Malnutrition in Children under Five and School Age Children in Low and Middle Income Countries (**Nemer L, Gelband H, Stansfield S, Jha P**)

Paper 12: Addressing the Impact of Household Energy and Indoor Air Pollution on the Health of the Poor – Implications for Policy Action and Intervention Measures (**Von Schirnding Y, Bruce N, Smith K, Ballard-Tremeer G, Ezzati M, Lvovsky K**)

Paper 13: Constraints to Scaling Up Health Interventions: A Conceptual Framework and Empirical Analysis (**Hanson K, Ranson MK, Oliveira Cruz V, Mills A**)

Paper 14: Approaches Overcoming Health Systems Constraints at the Peripheral Level: A Review of the Evidence (**Olivera Cruz V, Hanson K, Mills A**)

Paper 15: Constraints to Scaling Up Health Interventions: Country Case Study: India (**Rao Seshadri S**)

Paper 16: Constraints to Scaling Up Health Interventions: Country Case Study: Tanzania (**Munishi G**)

Paper 17: Constraints to Scaling Up Health Interventions: Country Case Study: Chad (**Wyss K, Moto DD, Callewaert B**)

Paper 18: Costs of Scaling Up Priority Health Interventions in Low-Income and selected Middle-Income Countries: Methodology and Estimates (**Kumaranayake L, Kurowski C, Conteh L**)

Paper 19: Study on Costs of Scaling Up Health Interventions for the Poor in Latin American Settings: Final Report (**Bertozzi S, Zurita V, Cahuana L, Corcho A, Rely K, Aracena B**)

Paper 20: Indirect Estimates of Avoidable Mortality in Low Income and Middle Income Countries (**Nguyen S, Jha P, Yu S, Paccaud F**)

Paper 21: Note on the Health Impact of Water and Sanitation Services (**Vaz LME, Jha P**)

Paper 22: Constraints to the Scale-Up of Priority Interventions Factoring in Quality of Governance and Policy Framework (**Vergin H**)

Paper 23: HIV/AIDS Control in India – Lessons from Tamil Nadu (**Ramasundaram S, Allaudin K, Charles B, Gopal K, Krishnamurthy P, Poornalingam R, Warren D**)

Paper 24: Preliminary Estimates of the Cost of Expanding TB, Malaria and HIV/AIDS Activities for Sub-Saharan Africa (**Kumaranayake L, Conteh L, Kurowski C, Watts C**)

Paper 25: The Evidence Base of Interventions in the Care and Management of AIDS in Low and Middle Income Countries (**Willbond B, Thottingal P, Kimani J, Vaz LME, Plummer F**)

Working Group 6

Paper 1: Development Assistance for Health (DAH): Average Commitments 1997–1999 (**Michaud C**)

Paper 2: Perspectives on Improving Health in Poor Countries: Qualitative Assessment of Multilateral Agency Views and Behaviour (**Nelson J**)

Paper 3: Ideas Work Better than Money in Generating Reform – But How? Assessing Efficiency of Swedish Development Assistance in Health to Vietnam (**Jerve AM**)

Paper 4: Qualitative Assessment of Bilateral Agency Views and Behaviour: Interviews With Non-Health Specialists (**Ojermark M**)

Paper 5: Global Health Initiatives and National Level Health Programs: Assuring Compatibility and Mutual Re-Enforcement (**Forsberg BC**)

Paper 6: Structural Adjustment and Health: A Literature Review of the Debate, its Role-Players and Presented Empirical Evidence (**Breman A, Shelton C**)

Paper 7: A Case Study on the European Commission's Contribution to Development Assistance and Health (DAH) (**Daniels D**)

Paper 8: Review of Externally Aided Projects in the Context of their Integration into the Health Service Delivery in Karnataka (**Narayan R**)

Paper 9: Notes on DAH and Its Effectiveness: The Interests of Recipient Countries (**Issaka-Tinorgah A**)

Paper 10: Recent Trends in Development Assistance in Health (**OECD**)

Appendix 2: ANALYSIS OF THE COSTS OF SCALING UP PRIORITY HEALTH INTERVENTIONS IN LOW- AND SELECTED MIDDLE-INCOME COUNTRIES[1]

PURPOSE

The purpose of this appendix is to present a brief description of the methodology and an analysis of the estimated costs of scaling up priority interventions. This analysis builds on the cost analysis undertaken for Working Group 5; a more detailed discussion of methodology for the close-to-client (CTC) level costs of the priority set of interventions is presented in the costing background paper.[2] There are two sections to this appendix. In the first section, an analysis of the cost results is undertaken by country income classification. This analysis estimates the total health expenditures required for reaching target levels of coverage, the amount of domestic resources for health that may be mobilized, and the net financing gap. In the second section, analyses are undertaken on a regional level.

ANALYSIS BY DEVELOPMENT ASSISTANCE COMMITTEE–BASED INCOME CLASSIFICATION AND DISEASE CLASSIFICATION

Incremental Cost Analysis (Main Analysis for WG5 Report): CTC-level costs of selected set of priority interventions

The cost analysis estimates the cost of scaling up the coverage of 49 priority health interventions (and 65 treatment lines) at the CTC level in 83 poor countries. These interventions have been identified as key in addressing the major health conditions among the poor (and are described in Table A2.A). The expansion of these activities is based on reaching target levels of coverage for 2007 and 2015, relative to estimates of coverage levels in the year 2002. The incremental cost analysis focuses on selected interventions at a CTC level, and so does not include all the services needed for the expansion of the entire local health system. The analysis assesses the full economic price of providing services. Costs include capital components and related requirements for complementary management and institutional support, as well as the investments in training new personnel and expanding facilities in order to deliver services at these higher levels of coverage.

The cost analysis was designed to estimate the volume of additional or *incremental* resources that would be required for a large-scale expansion of activities from existing levels of services. The costs of expanding activities are presented as the cost additional to current levels of health expenditure. Thus these costs estimates reflect the *additional* expenditure, which is required over and above current patterns of expenditure.

The costs of expanding services will vary by country according to the extent and type of illness, and also by demographic and socioeconomic factors. Hence the costs of scaling up have been modeled on a country-specific basis for each intervention, taking into account complementarities between interventions. *Poor countries* have been defined as those having a GNP per capita of less than US $1,200 (year 1999 US$). Given the substantial disease burden in sub-Saharan Africa, all countries of this region have been included in the analysis, independent of their economic performance.[3]

The costs of expanding services were prepared for two scenarios (see Working Group 5 Synthesis Paper), based on the level of investment and ability to expand services, reflecting different assumptions about the time-frame, investments in capacity and infrastructure, and feasible levels of target coverage required to achieve health benefits. The scenario presented here for 2007 assumes scaling up in the context of large-scale investments at both the peripheral and local-hospital levels, but is restricted by the extent to which these investments can take place within 5 years. The Commission endorses this scenario as the basis of its recommendations. Scenario 2015 assumes scaling up given large-scale investments over a period of 13 years to high levels of coverage for all interventions.

A model was used to estimate the cost of implementing the interventions, the required new investments in training staff and facilities, and the required management and institutional support. In order to obtain estimates of the costs of scaling up, first available demographic, behavioral, and epidemiological data are used to determine the size of the relevant target groups that the prevention and care interventions are designed to reach, in other words, the population in need (PIN). Second, estimates were made of the current level of coverage for these interventions. Target coverage levels for the interventions were also established (see Table 7 in text). Third, cost data drawn from a range of interventions were related to the size of the PIN in order to provide national estimates for each country. As we were doing a country-specific approach to estimating costs, in order to make the costs comparable, nontraded components of costs were adjusted for purchasing-power parity. Given the uncertainty regarding the need of services and the costs of different interventions, a likely low–high range of costs was estimated. Costs for required investments in training and facilities were calculated on the size of the PIN for each scenario based on contact time with health service staff and use of inpatient or ambulatory facilities. The management and institutional support component of the costs included administrative and support functions, monitoring, supervision, and institutional strengthening within the CTC level. These costs were also based on the size of the PIN.

The incremental costs estimates provide an *annual average* cost of implementing these activities in year 2002 constant US dollars.[4] These estimates have also been translated into projected budget flows on annual basis.

Estimation of the country-specific population in need for a particular service rests principally on two parameters: the population size and the incidence or prevalence of a condition or risk. Current estimates and future prospects of the population size are available. However, country-specific information on current morbidity or risks is limited. Due to this substantial lack of data, the incidence and prevalence of disease or risk have been assumed to be constant over time. Consequently, this approach ignores any potential changes in disease prevalence or incidence and any effect of the increased service coverage on patterns of disease. Whereas this is of little or no relevance for conditions such as obstructed labor, it is a more severe limitation for transmittable diseases, in particular HIV/AIDS and tuberculosis where an impact would be expected. There may also be increases in the incidence or prevalence of these diseases over time, however, and so the direction of the bias attributable to the assumption of constant incidence or prevalence is not clear.

Table A2.1 presents the estimates of the incremental cost package for all disease and condition groups, in terms of total dollars, per capita figures, and percent of GNP. Per capita figures were calculated on the basis of projected population estimates for the years 2007 and 2015.[5] GNP figures were estimated by assuming between 1 percent and 5 percent annual growth for per capita GNP.[6] The average cost estimate of the low–high range is presented.

Table A2.1. ANNUAL INCREMENTAL COSTS (US$ 2002) BY DEVELOPMENT ASSISTANCE
COMMITTEE-BASED INCOME CLASSIFICATION

	2007 Average Estimate	2015 Average Estimate
TOTAL DOLLARS ('000 000 000, BILLIONS OF DOLLARS)		
All countries	26	46
All Low-Income Countries	19	33
(Least-Developed Countries + Other Low-Income Countries)		
Least-Developed Countries	8	15
Other Low-Income Countries	11	18
Low-Middle-Income Countries	5	11
Upper-Middle-Income Countries	1	2
PER CAPITA ($)		
All countries	6	10
All Low-Income Countries	7	10
(Least-Developed Countries + Other Low-Income Countries)		
Least-Developed Countries	11	16
Other Low-Income Countries	5	8
Low-Middle-Income Countries	4	7
Upper-Middle-Income Countries	26	44
Percent of GNP		
All countries	0.7	0.9
All Low-Income Countries	1.3	1.6
(Least-Developed Countries + Other Low-Income Countries)		
Least-Developed Countries	3.4	4.5
Other Low-Income Countries	0.9	1.1
Low-Middle-Income Countries	0.3	0.4
Upper-Middle-Income Countries	0.6	0.9

Analysis by Health Condition

The set of interventions chosen have been broadly characterized by disease
or condition type (see Table A2.A), but in reality, the nature of health service delivery means that there are overlaps between them. For example,
malaria prophylaxis for pregnant women could be included under either
malaria prevention or maternity-related interventions. The latter was chosen, as this was the nature of the delivery mechanism. The analysis in
Table A2.2 shows the breakdown of incremental costs by health condition.

Whereas methods exist to attribute the burden of disease to specific illnesses or health problems, the practical implementation of most programs for these conditions cannot be considered separately within a health system. Achieving widespread coverage for these key programs will require substantial strengthening and upgrading throughout the existing health system, providing externality benefits for nonpriority health conditions. Although theoretically it is possible to cost each key intervention

Table A2.2. ANNUAL INCREMENTAL COSTS ($US 2002) BY HEALTH CONDITION

	2007 Average Estimate	2015 Average Estimate
TOTAL DOLLARS ('000 0000, BILLIONS OF DOLLARS)		
All interventions	26	46
TB Treatment	0.5	1
Malaria Prevention	2	3
Malaria Treatment	0.5	1
HIV Prevention	6	8
HIV Care	3	6
HIV Treatment (HAART)	5	8
Childhood-related illness – Treatment	4	11
Childhood-related illnesses – Immunization	1	1
Maternity-related illnesses	4	5
PER CAPITA ($)		
All interventions	5.9	9.5
TB Treatment	0.1	0.2
Malaria Prevention	0.5	0.7
Malaria Treatment	0.1	0.2
HIV Prevention	1.5	1.7
HIV Care	0.6	1.3
HIV Treatment (HAART)	1.2	1.7
Childhood-related illness – Treatment	0.9	2.2
Childhood-related illnesses – Immunization	0.2	0.3
Maternity-related illnesses	0.8	1.1
Percent of GNP		
All interventions	0.71	0.88
TB Treatment	0.02	0.02
Malaria Prevention	0.06	0.07
Malaria Treatment	0.01	0.02
HIV Prevention	0.18	0.16
HIV Care	0.08	0.12
HIV Treatment (HAART)	0.14	0.15
Childhood-related illness – Treatment	0.10	0.21
Childhood-related illnesses – Immunization	0.03	0.02
Maternity-related illnesses	0.10	0.11

Note: Smoking-control policies are included, but are assumed to be self-financing.

separately, in reality, the implementation of most programs must be considered and costed within the context of a health system.

Further adjustments were made to the incremental costs in order to reflect the costs of the process of scaling up (Table A2.3). These additional costs were done on a country-specific health system basis, so it would be misleading to attempt to undertake the same adjustment by health condition. Hence subsequent tables present totals for all interventions.

Adjustments to Reflect Requirements for the Process of Scaling Up
In addition to the costs of scaling-up interventions at the CTC level, the process of scaling up itself will require a range of other forms of support to ensure effective implementation. Four adjustments were undertaken to reflect additional expenditures beyond the incremental scaling up of this selected set of interventions.

First, a management cost above the CTC level was estimated based on total incremental costs, to reflect the necessary input from institutions above the CTC level (e.g., Ministry of Health) in the implementation of the scaled-up interventions. It was estimated that above-CTC management costs would be approximately 15 percent of the total incremental cost.

Second, it was assumed that an additional 15 percent would be required to improve absorptive capacity given the magnitude of resources required to scale up. This would include ensuring adequate financial and monitoring systems at both the district and above-district levels.

Third, the costs in Table A2.1 assume that existing levels of coverage are constant and adequate. In reality, the quality of existing coverage is highly variable. We thus made an adjustment in the costs to reflect the fact that it would be necessary to undertake expenditures to improve quality (e.g., ensuring adequate supply of drugs) for current levels of coverage. Thus the estimated expenditures for 2002 for the selected set of interventions were multiplied by a quality adjustment factor. This adjustment ranged from 10 percent to 25 percent of estimated 2002 expenditures, depending on the income level of the country. Fourth, public-sector wages are generally too low to attract staff and ensure good performance, as reflected in high attrition rates (for example to the private sector) and poor motivation. Moreover, scaling up will require recruitment of additional health-sector personnel. In order to adjust salaries to the level that might be needed to attract and retain staff, a 100 percent increase in salaries for all staff was factored in. This salary adjustment was made for all health-sector personnel, not just those who are additionally required for scaling up the interventions in the incremental package. Table A2.3 provides the estimates for the adjusted package by total dollars, per capita and percent of GNP.

Total Health Expenditure Required

In order to estimate total health expenditure required, a distinction was made between domestic health expenditure and donor expenditure in the form of ODA. Data were available on the extent of ODA spent in health for the 1997 to 1999 period, and it was assumed that this reflected the average in 1998.[7] It was also assumed that between 1998 and 2002, ODA

Table A2.3. INCREMENTAL ANNUAL COSTS ADJUSTED FOR SCALING-UP PROCESS ($US 2002) BY DEVELOPMENT ASSISTANCE COMMITTEE–BASED CLASSIFICATION

	2007 Average Estimate	2015 Average Estimate
TOTAL DOLLARS ('000 000 000, BILLIONS OF DOLLARS)		
All countries	57	94
All Low-Income Countries (Least-Developed Countries + Other Low-Income Countries)	40	66
Least-Developed Countries	17	29
Other Low-Income Countries	23	37
Low-Middle-Income Countries	14	24
Upper-Middle-Income Countries	3	4
PER CAPITA ($)		
All countries	13	20
All low-income countries (Least-Developed Countries + Other Low-Income Countries)	14	21
Least-Developed Countries	22	32
Other Low-Income Countries	12	17
Low-Middle-Income Countries	9	15
Upper-Middle-Income Countries	57	91
Percent of GNP		
All countries	1.6	1.8
All Low-Income Countries (Least-Developed Countries + Other Low-Income Countries)	2.7	3.3
Least-Developed Countries	6.9	8.8
Other Low-Income Countries	1.9	2.2
Low-Middle-Income Countries	0.7	0.8
Upper-Middle-Income Countries	1.3	1.8

in the health sector grew at an annual rate of 5 percent. Total health expenditure in 1999 was calculated based on the 1999 total health expenditure as a percentage of GNP.[8] By subtracting the ODA component from 1999 total health expenditure, total domestic resources spent on health in 1999 were estimated. Total health expenditure in 2002 was then estimated as the sum of estimated ODA flows in 2002 and domestic resources in 2002. The latter was derived by using the 1999 share of domestic resources relative to 1999 GNP and multiplying by 2002 GNP.

Total health expenditure required in 2007 and 2015 was then estimated as addition of the total health expenditure in 2002 and the scale-adjusted costs from Table A2.3. Table A2.4 presents the estimates for total

Table A2.4. REQUIRED ANNUAL TOTAL HEALTH EXPENDITURE BY DEVELOPMENT ASSISTANCE COMMITTEE–BASED CLASSIFICATION ($US 2002)

	2002 Baseline	2007 Average Estimate	2015 Average Estimate
TOTAL DOLLARS ('000 000 000, BILLIONS OF DOLLARS)			
All countries	106.1	162.8	200.3
All Low-Income Countries (Least-Developed Countries + Other Low-Income Countries)	53.3	93.5	119.3
Least-Developed Countries	8.5	25.3	37.2
Other Low-Income Countries	44.8	68.2	82.1
Low-Middle-Income Countries	41.1	55.0	65.1
Upper-Middle-Income Countries	11.7	14.3	16.0
PER CAPITA ($)			
All countries	26	38	42
All Low-Income Countries (Least-Developed Countries + Other Low-Income Countries)	21	34	38
Least-Developed Countries	13	34	41
Other Low-Income Countries	24	34	37
Low-Middle-Income Countries	28	36	40
Upper-Middle-Income Countries	266	315	339
Percent of GNP			
All countries	3.7	4.5	3.9
All Low-Income Countries (Least-Developed Countries + Other Low-Income Countries)	4.4	6.3	5.9
Least-Developed Countries	4.3	10.4	11.4
Other Low-Income Countries	4.4	5.5	4.9
Low-Middle-Income Countries	2.8	2.9	2.2
Upper-Middle-Income Countries	6.8	7.3	6.8

Table A2.5. POTENTIAL DOMESTIC RESOURCE MOBILIZATION ($US 2002) BY
DEVELOPMENT ASSISTANCE COMMITTEE–BASED CLASSIFICATION

	2002 Baseline	2007 Average Estimate	2015 Average Estimate
TOTAL DOLLARS ('000 000 000, BILLIONS OF DOLLARS)			
All countries	102.8	163.6	283.5
All Low-Income Countries	50.5	76.5	124.0
(Least-Developed Countries + Other Low-Income Countries)			
Least-Developed Countries	7.1	11.1	18.2
Other Low-Income Countries	43.4	65.5	105.8
Low-Middle-Income Countries	40.6	71.9	138.7
Upper-Middle-Income Countries	11.7	15.2	20.7
PER CAPITA ($)			
All countries	25	38	59
All Low-Income Countries	20	28	40
(Least-Developed Countries + Other Low-Income Countries)			
Least-Developed Countries	11	15	20
Other Low-Income Countries	23	32	47
Low-Middle-Income Countries	28	47	86
Upper-Middle-Income Countries	265	335	441
Percent of GNP			
All countries	3.6	4.6	5.5
All Low-Income Countries	4.1	5.1	6.1
(Least-Developed Countries+ Other Low-Income Countries)			
Least-Developed Countries	3.5	4.6	5.6
Other Low-Income Countries	4.3	5.3	6.3
Low-Middle-Income Countries	2.8	3.8	4.7
Upper-Middle-Income Countries	6.8	7.8	8.8

Note: *Assumes 1 percent of GNP increase in domestic resources for health in 2007 and 2 percent increase of GNP in 2015, compared with 2002 baseline. If this increment is greater than the amount needed for scaling up, then the country is assumed to mobilize the actual amount needed.*

health expenditure required annually, in order to achieve the 2007 and 2015 target coverage levels.

Analysis of Net Financing Gap for Increased Domestic Resource Mobilization

The net financing gap is calculated for the cost of scaling up these priority health interventions. In this analysis, it is assumed that there will be a 1 percent increase in the percentage of health expenditure relative to GNP due to increased domestic resource mobilization in 2007. It is assumed that, by 2015, the percentage of health expenditure relative to GNP has increased by 2 percent. The estimated level of domestic resource mobilization is provided in Table A2.5 for the years 2002, 2007, and 2015. The net financing gap estimates are presented in Table A2.6. This analysis is undertaken for each country, and then the results are aggregated for each income category. If the country's own domestic resources are greater than total health expenditures, we assume that the financing gap is exactly 0. If

Table A2.6. ANNUAL NET FINANCING GAP ($US 2002; DEVELOPMENT ASSISTANCE COMMITTEE–BASED CLASSIFICATION)

	2007 Average Estimate	2015 Average Estimate
TOTAL DOLLARS ('000 000 000, BILLIONS OF DOLLARS)		
All countries	22.1	30.7
All Low-Income Countries	20.5	28.4
(Least-Developed Countries+ Other Low-Income Countries)		
Least-Developed Countries	14.3	20.8
Other Low-Income Countries	6.2	7.5
Low-Middle-Income Countries	1.5	2.3
Upper-Middle-Income Countries	0.04	0
PER CAPITA ($)		
All countries	5	6
All Low-Income Countries	7	4
(Least-Developed Countries + Other Low-Income Countries)		
Least-Developed Countries	19	23
Other Low-Income Countries	3	3
Low-Middle-Income Countries	1	1
Upper-Middle-Income Countries	1	0
Percent of GNP		
All countries	0.6	0.6
All Low-Income Countries	1.4	1.4
(Least-Developed Countries + Other Low-Income Countries)		
Least-Developed Countries	5.9	6.4
Other Low-Income Countries	0.5	0.4
Low-Middle-Income Countries	0.1	0.1
Upper-Middle-Income Countries	0.02	0

Note: This analysis has been done on a country-specific basis and then summarized by the DAC grouping of countries. Thus, countries whose domestic resources are greater than their required health expenditures were treated as having a net financing gap of 0. If the required health expenditure is greater than domestic resources, their difference was included as a net financing gap for the country. Thus entries in Table A2.6 are not equal to the entries in Table A2.4 minus the entries in Table A2.5, as not every country had a in the DAC category has a positive net financing gap.

Table A2.7. INCREMENTAL ANNUAL COSTS ($US 2002) BY REGION

	2007 Average Estimate	2015 Average Estimate
TOTAL DOLLARS ('000 000 000, BILLIONS OF DOLLARS)		
All countries	26	46
Sub-Saharan Africa -low	10	18
Sub-Saharan Africa -mid	2	3
East Asia and Pacific	6	11
South Asia	7	11
Eastern Europe and Central Asia	0.4	0.8
Latin and Central America	0.4	0.8
PER CAPITA ($)		
All countries	6	10
Sub-Saharan Africa -low	14	21
Sub-Saharan Africa -mid	26	46
East Asia and Pacific	3	5
South Asia	5	7
Eastern Europe and Central Asia	4	7
Latin and Central America	9	16
Percent of GNP		
All countries	0.7	0.9
Sub-Saharan Africa -low	4.0	5.5
Sub-Saharan Africa -mid	0.8	1.2
East Asia and Pacific	0.3	0.3
South Asia	0.8	0.9
Eastern Europe and Central Asia	0.4	0.7
Latin and Central America	0.9	1.3

the country's own domestic resources are *less* than total health expenditures, the financing gap is the difference between the two. After calculating the financing gap on a country-by-country basis, these gaps are then aggregated across DAC categories in Table A2.6. Because of this method of calculation, the entries in Table A2.6 are not equal to the entries in Table A2.4 minus the entries in Table A2.5. This would be the case only if every country in the DAC category had a positive net financing gap.

ANALYSIS OF COST ESTIMATES BY REGION

This section presents data by regional classification. Table A2.C in the Appendix shows the grouping of countries by region. Tables A2.7 and A2.8 show the incremental and scale-adjusted costs by region. Table A2.8 presents an analysis of domestic resource mobilization, similar to the scenarios in Table A2.4. Tables A2.9 and A2.10 show the total health expenditures by region, and the net financing gap by region.

Table A2.8.   INCREMENTAL ANNUAL COSTS ADJUSTED FOR SCALING-UP PROCESS ($US 2002) BY REGION

	2007 Average Estimate	2015 Average Estimate
TOTAL DOLLARS ('000 000 000, BILLIONS OF DOLLARS)		
All countries	57	94
Sub-Saharan Africa -low	20	35
Sub-Saharan Africa -mid	4	7
East Asia and Pacific	15	25
South Asia	15	24
Eastern Europe and Central Asia	1	2
Latin and Central America	1	2
PER CAPITA ($)		
All countries	13	20
Sub-Saharan Africa -low	28	41
Sub-Saharan Africa -mid	56	91
East Asia and Pacific	8	13
South Asia	10	14
Eastern Europe and Central Asia	9	14
Latin and Central America	21	33
Percent of GNP		
All countries	1.6	1.8
Sub-Saharan Africa -low	8.1	10.7
Sub-Saharan Africa -mid	1.7	2.5
East Asia and Pacific	0.7	0.8
South Asia	1.7	1.9
Eastern Europe and Central Asia	1.0	1.4
Latin and Central America	2.0	2.8

Table A2.9. REQUIRED ANNUAL TOTAL HEALTH EXPENDITURE ($US 2002) BY REGION

	2002 Baseline	2007 Average Estimate	2015 Average Estimate
TOTAL DOLLARS ('000 00 0000, BILLIONS OF DOLLARS)			
All countries	106.1	162.8	200.3
Sub-Saharan Africa -low	8.3	28.6	43.7
Sub-Saharan Africa -mid	12.6	16.4	19.5
East Asia and Pacific	42.3	57.4	67.1
South Asia	36.0	51.4	59.8
Eastern Europe and Central Asia	4.5	5.5	6.2
Latin and Central America	2.5	3.4	4.1
PER CAPITA ($)			
All countries	26	38	42
Sub-Saharan Africa -low	13	40	50
Sub-Saharan Africa -mid	192	237	259
East Asia and Pacific	24	31	34
South Asia	25	34	35
Eastern Europe and Central Asia	39	47	50
Latin and Central America	60	76	82
Percent of GNP			
All countries	3.7	4.5	3.9
Sub-Saharan Africa -low	3.9	11.4	13.2
Sub-Saharan Africa -mid	6.4	7.3	7.0
East Asia and Pacific	2.7	2.8	2.1
South Asia	4.9	5.7	4.8
Eastern Europe and Central Asia	5.0	5.5	5.0
Latin and Central America	6.3	7.4	6.9

Table A2.10. ANNUAL DOMESTIC RESOURCE MOBILIZATION ($US 2002) BY REGION

	2002 Baseline	2007 Average Estimate	2015 Average Estimate
TOTAL DOLLARS ('000 00 0000, BILLIONS OF DOLLARS)			
All countries	102.8	163.6	283.5
Sub-Saharan Africa -low	7.0	10.8	17.5
Sub-Saharan Africa -mid	12.5	16.5	22.9
East Asia and Pacific	41.8	75.0	145.3
South Asia	34.9	52.3	84.8
Eastern Europe and Central Asia	4.4	5.9	8.4
Latin and Central America	2.2	3.0	4.5
PER CAPITA ($)			
All countries	25	38	59
Sub-Saharan Africa -low	11	15	20
Sub-Saharan Africa -mid	191	238	305
East Asia and Pacific	24	40	74
South Asia	25	34	50
Eastern Europe and Central Asia	38	51	69
Latin and Central America	53	68	89
Percent of GNP			
All countries	3.6	4.6	5.5
Sub-Saharan Africa -low	3.3	4.3	5.3
Sub-Saharan Africa -mid	6.3	7.3	8.2
East Asia and Pacific	2.6	3.6	4.6
South Asia	4.8	5.8	6.8
Eastern Europe and Central Asia	4.9	5.9	6.9
Latin and Central America	5.6	6.6	7.6

Table A2.11. ANNUAL NET FINANCING GAP ($US 2002) BY REGION

	2007 Average Estimate	2015 Average Estimate
TOTAL DOLLARS ('000 000 000, BILLIONS OF DOLLARS)		
All countries	22.1	30.7
Sub-Saharan Africa -low	17.8	26.2
Sub-Saharan Africa -mid	0.9	1.3
East Asia and Pacific	1.0	1.3
South Asia	1.7	1.4
Eastern Europe and Central Asia	0.2	0.2
Latin and Central America	0.5	0.2
PER CAPITA ($)		
All countries	5	6
Sub-Saharan Africa -low	25	30
Sub-Saharan Africa -mid	12	17
East Asia and Pacific	1	1
South Asia	1	1
Eastern Europe and Central Asia	2	2
Latin and Central America	12	5
Percent of GNP		
All countries	0.6	0.6
Sub-Saharan Africa -low	7.1	7.9
Sub-Saharan Africa -mid	0.4	0.5
East Asia and Pacific	0.05	0.04
South Asia	0.2	0.1
Eastern Europe and Central Asia	0.2	0.2
Latin and Central America	1.1	0.4

Note: This analysis has been done on a country-specific basis and then summarized by region. Thus, countries whose domestic resources are greater than their required health expenditures were treated as having a net financing gap of 0. If the required health expenditure is greater than domestic resources, their difference was included as a net financing gap for the country. Thus entries in Table A2.11 are not equal to the entries in Table A2.9 minus the entries in Table A2.10, as not every country in the region has a positive net financing gap.

Table A2.A.   SELECTED SET OF INTERVENTIONS

Tuberculosis Treatment	Directly observed short-course treatment for smear-positive patients Directly observed short-course treatment for smear-negative patients
Malaria Prevention	Insecticide-treated nets Residual indoor spraying
Malaria Treatment	Treatment for clinical episodes of malaria
HIV/AIDS Prevention	Youth focused interventions Interventions working with sex workers and clients Condom social marketing and distribution Workplace interventions Strengthening of blood transfusion systems Voluntary counseling and testing Prevention of mother-to-child transmission Mass media campaigns Treatment for sexually transmitted diseases
HIV/AIDS Care	Palliative care Clinical management of opportunistic illnesses Prevention of opportunistic illnesses Home-based care
HIV/AIDS HAART	Provision of HAART
Childhood Disease–Related Interventions (Treatment)	Treatment of various conditions (acute respiratory infections, diarrhea, causes of fever, malnutrition, anemia)
Childhood Disease–Related Interventions (Immunization)	Vaccinations (BCG, OPV, DPT, Measles, Hepatitis B, HiB)
Maternity-Related Interventions	Antenatal care Treatment of complications during pregnancy Skilled birth attendance Emergency obstetric care Postpartum care (including family planning)

Note: Not all interventions have been scaled up in each country. Instead, the costs of scaling up include the interventions for each country that are epidemiologically appropriate. For example, malaria control measures are not included in countries where malaria does not significantly contribute to the burden of disease. Source: Kumaranayake L, Kurowski C, Conteh L. (2001). Costs of Scaling-up Priority Health Interventions in Low and Selected Middle Income Countries. Background Paper for Working Group 5 – Improving the Health Outcomes of the Poor, Commission on Macroeconomics and Health.

Table A2.B. CLASSIFICATION OF COUNTRIES BY DEVELOPMENT ASSISTANCE
COMMITTEE–BASED CATEGORIES[1]

Country	Country
Least-Developed Countries	Côte d'Ivoire
Afghanistan	Georgia
Angola	Ghana
Bangladesh	India
Benin	Indonesia
Bhutan	Kenya
Burkina Faso	Kyrgyzstan
Burundi	Mongolia
Cambodia	Nicaragua
Central African Republic	Nigeria
Chad	Pakistan
Comoros	Republic of Moldova
Dem. Republic of the Congo	Senegal
Eritrea	Tajikistan
Ethiopia	Turkmenistan
Gambia	Ukraine
Guinea	Uzbekistan
Guinea-Bissau	Viet Nam
Haiti	Zimbabwe
Lao People's Dem. Republic	**Lower-Middle-Income Countries**
Lesotho	Albania
Liberia	Bolivia
Madagascar	Cape Verde
Malawi	China
Mali	(excluding Hong Kong SAR
Mauritania	Cuba
Mozambique	Djibouti
Myanmar	Equatorial Guinea
Nepal	Guyana
Niger	Honduras
Rwanda	Maldives
Sierra Leone	Namibia
Somalia	Papua New Guinea
Sudan	Philippines
Togo	Samoa
Uganda	Solomon Islands
United Rep. of Tanzania	Sri Lanka
Yemen	Swaziland
Zambia	Syrian Arab Republic
Other Low-Income Countries	Vanuatu
Armenia	**Upper-Middle-Income Countries**
Azerbaijan	Botswana
Cameroon	Gabon
Congo	South Africa

1. *Countries not included in this table were not costed.*

Table A2.C.   REGIONAL CLASSIFICATION OF COUNTRIES

Sub-Saharan Africa* – Low Income (SSA Low):
Angola, Benin, Burkina Faso, Burundi, Cameroon, Central African Republic, Chad, Comoros, Congo, Côte d'Ivoire, Democratic Republic of the Congo, Eritrea, Ethiopia, Gambia, Ghana, Guinea, Guinea-Bissau, Kenya, Lesotho, Liberia, Madagascar, Malawi, Mali, Mauritania, Mozambique, Niger, Nigeria, Rwanda, Senegal, Sierra Leone, Somalia, Sudan, Togo, Uganda, United Republic of Tanzania, Yemen, Zambia, Zimbabwe

Sub-Saharan Africa* – Middle Income (SSA Mid):
Botswana, Cape Verde, Djibouti, Equatorial Guinea, Gabon, Namibia, South Africa, Swaziland, Syrian Arab Republic

East Asia and Pacific (EAP):
Cambodia, China (excluding Hong Kong SAR and Macao SAR), Democratic People's Republic of Korea, Indonesia, Lao People's Democratic Republic, Mongolia, Myanmar, Papua New Guinea, Philippines, Samoa, Solomon Islands, Vanuatu, Viet Nam

South Asia (SA):
Afghanistan, Bangladesh, Bhutan, India, Maldives, Nepal, Pakistan, Sri Lanka

Eastern Europe and Central Asia (EEC):
Albania, Armenia, Azerbaijan, Georgia, Kyrgyzstan, Republic of Moldova, Tajikistan, Turkmenistan, Ukraine, Uzbekistan

Latin and Central America (LAC):
Bolivia, Cuba, Guyana, Haiti, Honduras, Nicaragua

*We have grouped two middle-eastern countries, Syrian Arab Republic and Yemen, within the sub-Saharan African group.

NOTES

1. Prepared by Lilani Kumaranayake, Christoph Kurowski, and Lesong Conteh, London School of Hygiene and Tropical Medicine.

2. Kumaranayake, L., C. Kurowski, and L. Conteh (2001). *Costs of Scaling-up Priority Health Interventions in Low and Selected Middle Income Countries.* Background Paper for Working Group 5 – Improving the Health Outcomes of the Poor, Commission on Macroeconomics and Health.

3. These cost figures reflect the estimated costs of improving the coverage of program activities on a national scale, aggregated on the basis of the 1997 OECD DAC criteria for classifying countries: Least-developed countries (LDC), other low-income countries (OLIC), lower-middle-income countries (LMIC), and upper-middle-income-countries (UMIC). The criteria are found in the OECD, *Development Cooperation Report* (The DAC Journal) 2000. When the classification into which countries fall is compared with the most recent World Development Report (WDR) by the World Bank, there are a number of differences, as the WDR presents a low/middle-income country classification based on 1999 GNP figures. We have thus revised the 1997 DAC classification to reflect these changes, and the list of countries is provided in the Table A2.B.

4. An average annual inflation rate of 3.2 percent was used to derive constant US dollars in terms of 2002 prices.

5. Population projections were taken from *The World Population Prospects, 1998 Revision,* published by the UN Department of Social and Economic Affairs, Population Division.

6. The GNP data are taken from the *World Development Report 2000/2001* published by the World Bank. Note that the GNP figures for the Democratic People's Republic of Korea were not available. A 5 percent annual per capita GNP growth rates was assumed for China. A 3 percent annual per capita GNP growth rate was assumed for Bangladesh, Bhutan, India, Indonesia, Lao People's Democratic Republic, Sri Lanka, and Viet Nam. A 2 percent annual per capita GNP growth rate was assumed for Albania, Armenia, Azerbaijan, Bolivia, Botswana, Cambodia, Cameroon, Cape Verde, Congo, Côte d'Ivoire, Cuba, Gabon, Georgia, Ghana, Guyana, Honduras, Kyrgyzstan, Maldives, Mongolia, Nepal, Nicaragua, Pakistan, Papua New Guinea, Philippines, Republic of Moldova, Samoa, Solomon Islands, South Africa, Syrian Arab Republic, Tajikistan, Turkmenistan, Ukraine, Uzbekistan, and Vanuatu. A 1 percent annual per capita GNP growth rate was assumed for the remaining countries.

7. *DAC Report 2000* published by the OECD.

8. Data taken from *The World Health Report 2000* published by WHO.

REFERENCES

Abel-Smith, B. and A. Leiserson. 1978. *Poverty, Development, and Health Policy.* Geneva: World Health Organization (Albany, N.Y.: Sold by WHO Publications Centre).

Accelerated Access Initiative. See http://www.unaids.org/acc_access/index.html

Anderson, J., M. Maclean, and C. Davies. 1996. *Malaria Research: An Audit of International Activity.* London: Wellcome Trust.

Arhin-Tenkorang, D. 2000. *Mobilizing Resources for Health: The Case for User Fees Re-visited,* CMH Paper No. WG3: 1, 2000.

Arhin-Tenkorang, D. and G. Buckle, 2001. "Cost of Scaling up Provision of Primary and Secondary Health Care Services in Ghana," Unpublished.

Attaran, A. and L. Gillespie-White. 2001. "Do Patents Constrain Access to AIDS Treatment in Poor Countries: Antiretroviral Drugs in Africa," *Journal of the American Medical Association,* 2001: 286.

Barro, R. and X. Sala-I-Martin. 1995. *Economic Growth.* New York: McGraw-Hill, Inc.

Basch, P. F. 1999. *Textbook of International Health*, 2nd edition. Oxford University Press, New York.

Becker, G., T. Philipson, and R. Soares. 2001. "Growth and Mortality in Less Developed Nations." Unpublished manuscript, University of Chicago.

Bhargava, A. and J. Yu. 1997. "A Longitudinal Analysis of Infant and Child Mortality Rates in Developing Countries," *Indian Economic Review* 32: 141–151.

Bhargava, A., T. Dean, L. J. Jamison, and C. J. L. Murray. 2001. "Modeling the Effects of Health on Economic Growth," *Journal of Health Economics* 20 (2001) 423–440.

Bloom, David E., D. Canning, and B. Graham. 2001. "Health, Longevity, and Life-Cycle Savings," CMH Working Group Paper No. WG1: 9, 2001.

Bloom, D. E. and J. D. Sachs. 1998. "Geography, Demography, and Economic Growth in Africa." *Brookings Papers on Economic Activity* 2: 207–295. http://www.cid.harvard.edu/.

Culter, D. M. and E. Richardson. 1997. "Measuring the Health of the U.S. Population," *Brookings Papers: Microeconomics,* pp. 217–271.

Curtis, C. F. 2001. "The Mass Effect of Widespread Use of Insecticide-Treated Bednets in a Community," CMH Policy Memorandum. http://www.cid.harvard.edu/.

Economist. 2001. "The Worst Way to Lose Talent," The Economist, February 8.

Ettling, J. 1981. The Germ of Laziness. Rockefeller Philanthropy and Public Health in the New South. Cambridge, Massachusetts and London, England: Harvard University Press.

Evans, D., A. Tandon, C. J. L. Murray, and J. A. Lauer. 2001. "Comparative Efficiency of National Health Systems: Cross National Econometric Analysis," British Medical Journal 323 (11 August 2001).

Fang J. and Q. Xiong. 2001. "Financial Reform and Its Impact on Health Service in Poor Rural China," paper presented at the Conference on Financial Sector Reform in China, Harvard University, September 2001.

Feachem, R. 2001. "Globalization: From Rhetoric to Evidence." Editorial in Bulletin of the World Health Organization, Geneva, September 2001.

Fogel, R. W. 1991. "New Sources and New Techniques for the Study of Secular Trends in Nutritional Status, Health, Mortality and the Process of Aging." National Bureau of Economic Research Working Paper Series as Historical Factors and Long Run Growth, No. 26.

Fogel, R. W. 1997. "New Findings on Secular Trends in Nutrition and Mortality: Some Implications for Population Theory," in M. R. Rosenzweig and O. Stark (eds.), Handbook of Population and Family Economics, Vol. 1a. Amsterdam: Elsevier Science, pp. 433–481.

Fogel, R. W. 2000. The Fourth Great Awakening and the Future of Egalitarianism. Chicago and London: The University of Chicago Press.

Gallup, J. L. and J. D. Sachs. 2001. "The Economic Burden of Malaria," American Journal of Tropical Medicine and Hygiene Special Supplement, June.

Gertler, P. and J. Gruber. 2001. "Insuring Consumption Against Illness." Forthcoming in the American Economic Review.

Global Alliances for Vacines and Immunizations. 2001. "Global Immunization Challenges." Available at http://www.vaccinealliance.org/reference/globalimm-challenges.html)

Global Forum for Health Research. 1999. "The 10/90 Report on Health Research." Geneva: Global Forum for Health Research.

Gupta, S., M. Verhoeven, and E. Tiongson. 2001. "Public Spending on Health Care and the Poor," IMF Working Paper No. 01/127

Gwatkin, D. 2000a. "Poverty and Inequalities in Health within Developing Countries: Filling the Information Gap," in D. Leon and G. Walt, (eds), *Poverty, Inequality, and Health: An International Perspective*. Oxford: Oxford University Press, pp. 217–246.

Gwatkin, D. R. 2000b. "Health Inequalities and the Health of the Poor: What Do We Know? What Can We Do?" *Bulletin of the World Health Organization* 78 (1).

Gwatkin, D. R., S. Rutstein, K. Johnson, R. P. Pande, and A. Wagstaff. 2001. "Socio-Economic Differences in Health, Nutrition and Population" (a series of reports on 44 developing countries). Washington, DC: World Bank.

Hanson, K., K. Ranson, V. Oliveira, and A. Mills. 2001. "Constraints to Scaling Up Health Interventions: A Conceptual Framework and Empirical Analysis," CMH Working Paper Series No. WG5: 13. Available at http://www.cid.harvard.edu

Henry, B., S. Pollock, B. Kawa, B. Yaffe, F. Jamieson, E. Rea, and M. Avendano. 2000. "Tuberculosis Outbreak in Tibetan Refugee Claimants in Canada," presented at the 5th Annual Meeting of the International Union Against TB and Lung Disease, North American Region, Vancouver, February 2000. Available at http://www.hc-sc.gc.ca/hpb/lcdc/survlnce/fetp.

Hensher, M. 2001. "Financing Health Systems Through Efficiency Gains," CMH Working Paper Series No. WG3: 5. Available at http://www.cid.harvard.edu

Hirschler, B. 2001. "RPT-Glaxo Gives Up Rights to AIDS Drugs in South Africa," Reuters, October 8.

Huber, M. 1999. "Health Expenditure Trends in OECD Countries, 1970–1997," *Health Care Financing Review* 21(2).

IFMPA, Report of the WHO/IFPMA Round Table Discussions, 3 November 1999, Second WHO-IFPMA Round Table, WHO Headquarters, Geneva. Available at http://www.ifpma.org

IMF. 2001a. "Heavily Indebted Poor Countries (HIPC) Initiative: Status of Implementation," May 25. Available at http://www.imf.org/

IMF. 2001b. "Debt Relief for Poor Countries (HIPC): What Has Been Achieved," August. Available at http://www.imf.org/external/np/exr/facts/povdebt.htm

IMF. 2001c. *A Manual of Government Finance Statistics*. Washington, DC: International Monetary Fund.

IMF, OECD, UN, The World Bank. 2000. *Progress Towards the International Development Goals: 2000 A Better World for All*. Washington, DC.

Initiative on Public-Private Partnerships for Health (IPPPH), info@ippph.org

International Organization for Migration. 2001. *World Migration Report 2000*. Geneva: UN Publications.

Interim Working Group (IWG) on Reproductive Health Commodity Security. 2001. "Contraceptive Projections and the Donor Gap," Washington, DC: Interim Working Group (IWG) on Reproductive Health Commodity Security.

Jones, T. 1990. "The Panama Canal: A Brief History." Available at http://www.ilove-languages.com/Tyler/

Korber, B., M. Muldoon, J. Theiler, F. Gao, R. Gupta, A. Lapedes, B. H. Hahn, S. Wolinksy, and T. Bhattacharya. 2000. "Timing the Ancestor of the HIV-1 Pandemic Strains," *Science* 288: 1789–1796.

Kremer, M. and T. Miguel. 1999. "The Educational Impact of De-Worming in Kenya," paper presented at the Northeast Universities Development Conference held at Harvard University on October 8th and 9th.

Kremer, M. 2001. "Public Policies to Stimulate Development of Vaccines and Drugs for Neglected Diseases," CMH Paper No. WG2: 7, July.

Kumaranayake L., C. Kurowski, and L. Conteh. 2001 *Costs of Scaling-up Priority Health Interventions in Low and Selected Middle Income Countries*. Available at http://www.cid.harvard.edu

Lanjouw, J. 2001. "A Patent Policy Proposal for Global Diseases," *Brookings Policy Brief*, June.

Laver, G. and E. Garman. 2001. "The Origin and Control of Pandemic Influenza," *Science* 293 (7 September): 1776–1777.

Lewis, P.D., R. Balazs, A. J. Patel, and T. C. Jordan. 1986. "Undernutrition and Brain Development," in F. Falkner and J. M. Tanner, (eds.). *Human Growth*, 2nd edition. New York: Plenum Press, pp. 415–473.

Liu, Y. and W. Hsiao. 2001. "China's Poor and Poor Policy: The Case for Rural Health Insurance," presented at the Conference on Financial Sector Reform in China, Harvard University, 13 September.

Machekano, R., W. McFarland, V. Mzezewa, S. Ray, S. Mbizvo, M. Basset, A. Latif, P. Mason, L. Gwanzura, L. Moses, C. Ley, and B. Brown. 1998. "Peer Education Reduces HIV Infection among Factory Workers in Harare, Zimbabwe." Abstract No. 15, 5th Conference on Retroviruses and Opportunistic Infections, Chicago, Illinois.

Misra, R., R. Chaterjee, and S. Rao. 2001. "Changing the Indian Health System: Current Issues, Future Directions." Unpublished.

Murray, C. J. L. and A. D. Lopez, eds. 1996. *The Global Burden of Disease and Injury Series*. Vol. 1: *A Comprehensive Assessment of Mortality and Disability from Diseases, Injuries, and Risk Factors in 1990 and Projected to 2020*. Cambridge, Massachusetts: Published by the Harvard School of Public Health on behalf of the World Health Organization and the World Bank, Harvard University Press.

National Intelligence Council. 2000. "The Global Infectious Disease Threat and Its Implications for the United States," Washington, DC, January 2000. Available at http://www.cia.gov/

National Intelligence Council Report. 2000. "Global Trends 2015: A Dialogue with Non-Governmental Experts," December 2000. Available at http://www.cia.gov/.

OECD. 2000. *Development Cooperation Report* (The DAC Journal). Paris: Organisation for Economic Cooperation and Development.

Philipson, T. and R. Soares. 2001. "Human Capital, Longevity, and Economic Growth: A Quantitative Assessment of Full Income Measures." Working Paper, Washington DC: World Bank.

Pollitt, E. 2001. The Developmental and Probabilistic Nature of the Functional Consequences of Iron-Deficiency Anemia in Children," *The Journal of Nutrition.* 131: 669S–675S.

Pollitt, E. 1997. "Iron Deficiency and Educational Deficiency," *Nutritional Reviews* 55(4): 133–140.

Preker, A. 1998. "The Introduction of Universal Access to Health Care in OECD: Lessons for Developing Countries," in S. S. Nitayarumphong and A. Mills, (eds.). *Achieving Universal Coverage of Health Care: Experiences from Middle and Upper Income Countries.* Bangkok, Thailand: Ministry of Public Health, Office of Health Care Reform.

Preston, S. H. and M. R. Haines. 1991. *Fatal Years: Child Mortality in Late Nineteenth-Century America.* Princeton, N.J.: Princeton University Press.

Sachs, J. 2001. "The Strategic Significance of Global Inequality," *The Washington Quarterly*, Summer: 191.

Sen, A. 1999. *Development as Freedom.* New York: Alfred A. Knopf.

Simms, C., M. Rowson, and S. Peattie. 2001. "The Bitterest Pill of All: The Collapse of Africa's Health Care System," London: Save the Children UK.

Stanton, B. F., X. Li, J. Kahihuata, A. M. Fitzgerald, S. Neumbo, G. Kanduuombe, I. B. Ricardo, J. S. Galbraith, N. Terreri, I. Guevara, H. Shipena, J. Strijdom, R. Clemens, and R. F. Zimba. 1998. "Increased Protected Sex and Abstinence Among Namibian Youth Following a HIV Risk-Reduction Intervention: A Randomized, Longitudinal Study," *AIDS* 12: 2473–2480.

State Failure Task Force. 1999. "State Failure Task Force Report: Phase II Findings," in the *Environmental Change and Security Project Report* of the Woodrow Wilson Center, Issue 5, Summer: 49–72.

Strauss, J., and D. Thomas. 1998. "Health, Nutrition and Economic Development," *Journal of Economic Literature.* 36: 766–817.

Swedish International Development Agency (SIDA). 2001. "Global Health Initiatives and Poverty Reduction: Guiding Principles for Maximum Country-Level Impact," 10 April.

Thomas, D. and J. Strauss. 1997."Health and Wages: Evidence on Men and Women in Urban Brazil," *Journal of Econometrics* 77: 159–185.

Topel, R. and K. Murphy, 1997. "Unemployment and Nonemployment," *American Economic Review* 87 (May): 295–300.

"Transitional Arrangements" Report, meeting on the Global Fund to Fight AIDS, Tuberculosis, and Malaria (GFATM), Brussels, 12–13 July 2001.

Tucker, J. 2001. *Scourge.* New York: Atlantic Monthly Press.

United Nations. 2000. *We the peoples: The Role of the United Nations in the Twenty-First Century.* The Millennium Report, 2000. New York: United Nations.

United Nations Development Program. 1990. *Human Development Report, 1990: Concept and Measurement of Human Development.* New York/Oxford: Oxford University Press.

United Nations Development Program. 2001. *Human Development Report, 2001: Making Technology Work for Human Development.* New York/Oxford: Oxford University Press.

United Nations Department of Social and Economic Affairs, Population Division. 1998. *The World Population Prospects, 1998 Revision.* New York: UN Department of Social and Economic Affairs.

Wagstaff, A. 2000. *Research on Equity, Poverty and Health Outcomes: Lessons from the Developing World.* Washington, DC: Development Research Group and Human Development Network, The World Bank.

Widdus, R. 2001. "Public-Private Partnerships for Health," *Bulletin of the World Health Organization* 79(8): 713–720.

Wolfgang, M. 1997. *Prentice-Hall Encyclopedia of World Proverbs.* New York: Prentice Hall.

WHO International Consultative Meeting on HIV/AIDS Antiretroviral Therapy, WHO, Geneva, 22–23 May 2001.

WHO, UNICEF, UNAIDS, World Bank, UNESCO, and UNFPA. 2000. *Health, A Key to Prosperity: Success Stories in Developing Countries.* Geneva: World Health Organization.

Working Group 2 of the Commission on Macroeconomics and Health. 2001. "Global Public Goods for Health: New Strategies for the 21st Century," Synthesis Paper. Available at http://www.cid.harvard.edu

Workshop on Differential Pricing and Financing of Essential Drugs, organized by WHO and WTO, 8–11 April 2001, Hosbjor, Norway.

World Bank Group. 2000. *World Development Report 2000/2001: Attacking Poverty.* New York: Oxford University Press.

World Health Organization. 1999. *The World Health Report 1999: Making a Difference.* Geneva: World Health Organization.

World Health Organization. 2000. *The World Health Report 2000: Health Systems: Improving Performance.* Geneva: World Health Organization.

Working Group 5 of the Commission on Macroeconomics and Health. 2001. "Interventions, Constraints and Costs in Improving Health Outcomes of the Poor" Synthesis Report. Available at http://www.cid.harvard.edu

DATA SOURCES

USAID database

DFID database

DAC on-line database

Data provided by AfDB, IADB, WB, WHO, UNICEF, DFID, USAID

Data on donor funding provided by AfDB, ADB, IADB, WB, WHO, UNICEF, DFID, USAID OECD CRS database for all other bilateral agencies

POLICY MEMORANDUMS

Attaran, A. 2001. "Health as a Human Right," CMH Policy Memorandum No. 3. Available at http://www.cid.harvard.edu

Curtis, C. F. 2001 "The Mass Effect of Widespread Use of Insecticide-Treated Bednets in a Community," CMH Policy Memorandum No. 4. Available at http://www.cid.harvard.edu/.

Jamison, D. and J. Wang. 2001. "Female Life Expectancy in a Panel of Countries, 1975–90," CMH Policy Memorandum. Available at http://www.cid.harvard.edu.

GLOSSARY

ADB: Asian Development Bank: multilateral development finance institution, owned by 59 member states, dedicated to reducing poverty in Asia and the Pacific. See http://www.adb.org

AfDB: African Development Bank: Regional multilateral development bank, owned by 77 nations, engaged in promoting the economic development and social progress of its regional member countries through making loans and equity investments, providing technical assistance for the preparation and execution of development projects and programs, promoting investment of public and private capital for development purposes, and responding to requests for assistance in coordinating development policies and plans of its member countries. The bank is also required to give special attention to national and multinational projects and programs that promote regional integration. See http://www.afdb.org

African Sleeping Sickness: see trypanosomiasis.

ANC: Antenatel care: Health care in the period between conception and birth. Same as prenatal care.

ARI: Acute Respiratory Tract Infection.

ART: Anti-Retroviral Therapy is treatment with antiretroviral drugs. Antiretroviral drugs are medicines that prevent the reproduction of a type of virus called a retrovirus. These medicines are used to treat acquired immune deficiency syndrome (AIDS) because the human immunodeficiency virus (HIV) that causes the disease is a retrovirus. Antiretroviral drugs cannot cure HIV infections, but are able to minimize conditions caused by the virus, such as opportunistic infections that would otherwise be rapidly fatal.

BCG: Bacillus Calmette Guerin: A special strain of tubercle bacilli used as a vaccine against tuberculosis.

Bilateral agency: A bilateral agency is a governmental organization in a developed country that works directly with national organizations in developing countries, usually by providing assistance in areas such as health and education. Examples of bilateral agencies include the United States Agency for International Development (USAID),

Department for International Development (DFID), Swedish International Development Cooperation Agency (SIDA), and Canadian International Development Agency (CIDA).

Brain drain: The exodus of professionals from one country, normally in which socioeconomic indicators are low, to obtain improved economic and social status by working in another country.

CGIAR: Consultative Group on International Agricultural Research: association supporting agricultural research and other activities of an international public goods nature. CGIAR is composed of sixteen autonomous research centers and is co-sponsored by the World Bank, FAO, and UNDP. See http://www.cgiar.org

Chagas disease: A disease that is caused by infection with the parasite known as *Trypanosoma cruzi* Chagas, carried by insects or bugs known as *triatomine* or *kissing bugs*. These insects are very common in Central and South America, where they inhabit poorly constructed houses and huts. The disease involves damage to the nerves that control the heart and digestive and other organs, and eventually leads to damage to these organs. Worldwide, Chagas disease affects over 15 million persons and kills 50,000 each year. Researchers believe that the parasite that causes the disease is found only in the Americas.

COI study: Cost of illness study: A study that itemizes, values, and sums the costs of a particular health problem with the aim of giving an idea of its economic burden.

Community financing scheme: A scheme in which a community pools funds and shares risks, and that is constituted of payees and decision-makers/managers.

Compulsory licensing: Compulsory licensing is a provision within the TRIPS Agreement that developing nations can use to achieve access to patented drugs. It authorizes and provides the conditions under which a third party may make, use, or sell a patented invention without the patent owner's consent.

CRS: Congenital Rubella Syndrome: A condition in which the rubella virus passes from an infected pregnant mother to her baby that results in physical and mental disabilities in the baby.

CTC system: Close-to-client system: That part of the health system—including basic hospitals, health centers, and health posts—where care is provided to the community.

DAC: Development Assistance Committee of the OECD: The principal body through which the OECD deals with issues related to cooperation with developing countries. DAC "concentrates on how international development co-operation contributes to the capacity of developing countries to participate in the global economy and the capacity of people to overcome poverty and participate fully in their societies."

DAH: Development Assistance to Health: Financial aid provided to developing countries to support their health activities.

DALYs: Disability-Adjusted Life Years: A measure that considers the burden of a disease to a population in terms of years of lost life, adjusted for the effect on health to those living with the disease. The aim is for this "weighting" to take into account qualitative and subjective aspects of disease and health, and value judgments of the population on the relative importance of different aspects of morbidity.

Demographic transition: A theory that relates population change to levels of economic development, in which populations shift from a condition characterized by high birth and death rates to one characterized by low birth and death rates in response to improving standards of living. In the middle stage of transition, when death rates are low, but birth rates remain high, populations may expand rapidly for several decades or more.

DFID: Department for International Development, United Kingdom: British government department responsible for "promoting development and the reduction of poverty. Its central focus is a commitment to an internationally agreed target to halve the proportion of people living in extreme poverty by 2015. In addition, associated targets include ensuring basic health care provision and universal access to primary education by the same date." See http://www.dfid.gov.uk/

Differential pricing: The sale of the same commodity to different buyers at different prices.

Disease burden: A measure of the size of a health problem in an area. Knowledge of the burden of disease can help determine where investment in health should be targeted.

DOTS treatment: Directly Observed Treatment, Short-Course: A strategy used in the treatment of TB in which healthcare workers directly observe patients taking medication. The objective is to treat patients by directly observing them take their medication for at least the first two months. This is to ensure that medication is taken in the right combinations and appropriate dosage in an effort to control and reduce the incidence of multidrug-resistant TB. With direct observation of treatment, it is anticipated that 80 percent of deaths attributed to TB worldwide will be prevented.

DPT: A combination vaccine that protects against diphtheria, pertussis, and tetanus. In many developing countries, full vaccination against these diseases requires a course of three doses of the vaccine. Often the doses are referred to as DPT1, DPT 2, and DPT 3.

EPI: Expanded Program on Immunization: Program launched by the WHO in 1974 with the goal of immunizing the world's children against six target diseases: diphtheria, tetanus, whooping cough (also called pertussis), polio, measles, and tuberculosis.

Essential medicines: Essential drugs/medicines are those that satisfy the health care needs of the majority of the population; they should therefore be available at all times in adequate amounts and in the appropriate dosage forms, and at a price that individuals and the community can afford. Many of these drugs/medicines are too expensive for those in the developing world to buy. Other life-saving treatments are not available because manufacturers have abandoned their production because they were not considered profitable enough.

Faith-based groups: Organizations that provide welfare services under the Charitable Choice provision in The Personal Responsibility and Work Opportunity Reconciliation Act of 1996, which restricts the US federal government from infringing upon the religious nature of any organization administering welfare-related assistance. Under the law, these religious organizations retain their independence from all levels of government. For example, the law allows faith-based groups to discriminate on the basis of religion.

Fertility rate (total): The average number of children a woman will have during her lifetime. The total fertility rate in developing countries tends to be between two and seven; in industrial countries it is usually less than two.

Filariasis: Filariasis is caused by nematodes (roundworms) that inhabit the lymphatics and subcutaneous tissues. The major forms are lymphatic filariasis, also known as *elephantiasis* (caused by *Wuchereria bancrofti* and *Brugia malayi*), and onchocerciasis, also known as *river blindness* (caused by *onchocerca volvulus*). Lymphatic filariasis is transmitted by mosquito, affects an estimated 120 million persons throughout the tropics, and is ranked by the World Health

Organization (WHO) as the second leading cause of permanent disability worldwide. The nematodes responsible for onchocerciasis are carried by a blackfly that is found in fertile riverside areas. These areas are often deserted because of fear of the blindness. Onchocerciasis constitutes a serious obstacle to socioeconomic development.

GATT: General Agreement on Tariffs and Trade: The WTO's predecessor, the GATT, was established on a provisional basis after the Second World War in the wake of other new multilateral institutions dedicated to international economic cooperation—notably the Bretton Woods institutions now known as the World Bank and the International Monetary Fund. It served as the basis for the multilateral trading system from 1947 until the formation of the WTO on 1 January 1995.

GAVI: Global Alliance for Vaccines and Immunization: Alliance of multinational agencies, bilateral agencies, international development banks, foundations, pharmaceutical industry, NGOs, and government health programs formed in 1999 "to address flagging interest and to increase support for immunization."
See http://www.vaccinealliance.org

GEF: Global Environmental Facility: Facility established in 1991 to "forge international cooperation and finance actions to address four critical threats to the global environment: biodiversity loss, climate change, degradation of international waters, and ozone depletion."
See http://www.gefweb.org

GFATM: Global Fund to Fight AIDS, Tuberculosis, and Malaria: A fund established after the UN General Assembly Special Session on HIV/AIDS of June 2001. The fund is intended "to serve as a means for mobilizing, managing and disbursing new and additional resources to address the challenges created by the severe epidemics of TB and malaria and the serious threat posed by HIV/AIDS."

GHRF: Global Health Research Fund: A new fund for health research advocated by the Commission on Macroeconomics and Health. It is one of the major channels recommended by the Commission to increase health-related research and development, with disbursements of around $1.5 billion per year. This fund would support basic and applied biomedical and health sciences research on the health problems affecting the world's poor and on the health systems and policies and policies needed to address them. A key goal of the GHRF would

be to build long-term research capacity in developing countries themselves, by providing vital funding for research groups in low-income
countries.

GNP: Gross National Product: The value of a country's final output of
goods and services in a year. The value of GNP can be calculated by
adding up the amount of money spent on a country's final output of
goods and services, or by totaling the income of all citizens of a country including the income from factors of production used abroad.

GPGs: Global Public Goods: Goods whose characteristics of publicness
(nonrivalry in consumption and nonexcludability of benefits) extend
to more than one set of countries or more than one geographic
region.

HAART: Highly Active Anti-Retroviral Therapy: An antiretroviral regimen, employing a combination of antiretroviral drugs and used in
AIDS treatment, that can reasonably be expected to reduce the viral
load to <50 c/ml in treatment-naïve patients.

Healthy life years: A year of life in which the individual is free of health
problems.

HepB: Hepatitis B: Hepatitis is an "inflammation of the liver," which
can be caused by many things such as viruses, bacterial infections,
trauma, adverse drug reactions, or alcoholism. Hepatitis B is transmitted primarily through blood, unprotected sex, shared needles, and
from an infected mother to her newborn during the delivery process.

HIB/HiB: *Haemophilus influenzae* B: A frequent cause of bacterial
infections (e.g., meningitis, blood infections, pneumonia, arthritis) in
infants and young children.

HIC: High-income countries: Those countries with an annual per capita
GNP of more than $9,385 in 1995, as listed in the DAC List of Aid
Recipients used for the years 1997–1999.

HIPC Initiative: The Heavily Indebted Poor Countries Initiative is
described by the World Bank as its program whose principal objective
is to bring countries' debt burden to sustainable levels, subject to sat-
isfactory policy performance, so as to ensure that adjustment and
reform efforts are not put at risk by continued high debt and debt
service burdens. The Initiative involves an agreement among official
creditors to help the most heavily indebted countries to obtain debt
relief.

HIV/AIDS: Human Immunodeficiency Virus/Acquired Immune Deficiency Syndrome. The retrovirus isolated and recognized as the etiologic (ie, causing or contributing to the cause of a disease) agent of AIDS. AIDS is the most severe manifestation of infection with HIV. Persons living with AIDS often have infections of the lungs, brain, eyes, and other organs, and frequently suffer debilitating weight loss, diarrhea, and a type of cancer called Kaposi's Sarcoma.

HRP: Special Programme of Research, Development and Research Training in Human Reproduction. The Programme is a joint effort of UNDP/UNFPA/WHO/World Bank, and was established in 1972 by WHO. It continues to exist as an entity within the WHO Department of Reproductive Health and Research.

IADB: Inter-American Development Bank: Regional multilateral development institution with 46 member nations. The IADB was established in December of 1959 to "help accelerate economic and social development in Latin America and the Caribbean." See http://www.iadb.org

IBN: Insecticide-impregnated bednets: Bednets impregnated with insecticide. Studies have shown that in malaria-endemic areas, regular use of insecticide-impregnated bednets can reduce childhood mortality by 20 percent or more. Severe disease can be reduced by up to half.

IBRD: International Bank for Reconstruction and Development: An institution of the World Bank, providing loans and development assistance to middle-income countries and creditworthy poorer countries. See http://www.worldbank.org/ibrd/

IDA: International Development Association: Part of the World Bank that lends on highly concessional terms, providing long-term loans at zero interest and a low administrative fee to the poorest of the developing countries. The mission of IDA is to "support efficient and effective programs to reduce poverty and improve the quality of life in its poorest member countries." See http://www.worldbank.org/ida/

IFPMA: International Federation of Pharmaceutical Manufacturers Associations: A nonprofit, nongovernmental organization whose members are regional and national associations representing research-based pharmaceutical companies and other manufacturers of prescription medicines. The objectives of the Federation are to "deal with questions of common interest (eg, health legislation, science, research) in order to contribute to the advancement of the health and welfare of the peoples of the world; promote and support continuous development throughout the pharmaceutical industry of ethical principles and practices; to contribute expertise to and cooperation with national and international, governmental or nongovernmental, organisations with the same aims; coordinate the efforts of Members to meet these objectives." See http://www.ifpma.org

IMCI: Integrated Management of Childhood Illness: A strategy developed by WHO and UNICEF. "IMCI is an integrated approach to child health that focuses on the well-being of the whole child. IMCI aims to reduce death, illness and disability, and to promote improved growth and development among children under 5 years of age. IMCI includes both preventive and curative elements that are implemented by families and communities as well as by health facilities." See http://www.who.int/child-adolescent-health/integr.htm

IMR: Infant mortality rate: The number of infants, out of every 1,000 babies born in a given year, who die before reaching age 1. The lower the rate, the fewer the infant deaths, and generally the greater the level of health care available in a country.

ITN: Insecticide-treated mosquito net. See IBN.

IVR: Initiative for Vaccine Research: A WHO/UNAIDS initiative designed to bring the various vaccine research efforts of WHO and UNAIDS together, in order to streamline these activities, maximize synergies, and increase their focus. Its mission is to guide, enable, and facilitate the development, clinical evaluation, and worldwide access to safe, effective, and affordable vaccines against infectious diseases of public health importance, especially in developing countries.

LDC: Least-developed country: 1n 1997, the United Nations and the DAC List of Aid Recipients listed 48 countries as "least developed countries" (LDCs). The Economic and Social Council of the United Nations reviews the list every 3 years. A country qualifies to be added to the list of LDCs if it meets inclusion thresholds of three criteria: low income, as measured by the gross domestic product (GDP) per capita (in 2001, the threshold for low income is a per capita GDP of less than $800); weak human resources, as measured by a composite index (Augmented Physical Quality of Life Index) based on indicators of life expectancy at birth, per capita calorie intake, combined primary and secondary school enrollment, and adult literacy; and low level of economic diversification, as measured by a composite index (Economic Diversification Index) based on the share of manufacturing in GDP, the share of the labor force in industry, annual per capita commercial energy consumption, and United Nations Conference on Trade and Development merchandise export concentration index.

LEB: Life expectancy at birth: The average number of years newborn babies can be expected to live based on current health conditions. This indicator reflects environmental conditions in a country, the health of its people, the quality of care they receive when they are sick, and their living conditions.

Leishmaniasis: Leishmaniasis refers to several different illnesses caused by infection with an organism called a protozoan (simple single-celled organisms). The types of protozoa that cause leishmaniasis are carried by the blood-sucking sandfly. The course of the disease depends on the specific type of protozoa, and on the type of reaction the protozoa elicits from the patient's immune system. About 20 million people throughout the world are infected with leishmaniasis.

Leprosy: A chronic disease caused by infection with an acid-fast bacillus of the genus *Mycobacterium* (*M. leprae*). It is characterized by the formation of nodules on the surface of the body, especially on the face, or by the appearance of tuberculoid macules on the skin that are accompanied by loss of sensation. If untreated, it leads to involvement of nerves with eventual paralysis, wasting of muscle, and production of deformities and mutilations. In 2000, there were 680,000 registered cases and an estimated 1.6 million total cases of leprosy worldwide.

LIC: Low-income countries: Those countries with an annual per capita income of less than $765 in 1995, as listed in the DAC List of Aid Recipients used for the years 1997–1999. Under the DAC classification, LICs comprise both LDCs and OLICs.

LMIC: Lower-middle-income countries: LMIC countries have a Gross National Product per capita equivalent to more than $756 but less than $2,995 (1999). The standard of living in LMICs is higher than in low-income countries, and people have access to more goods and services, but many people still cannot meet their basic needs.

Lymphatic filariasis: Also known as *elephantiasis*. See filariasis.

Malaria: A tropical parasitic disease that kills more people than any other communicable disease except tuberculosis. Malaria is transmitted through the bite of an *Anopheles* mosquito, and, if promptly diagnosed and adequately treated, is curable. Symptoms include high fever, severe chills, enlarged spleen, repeated vomiting, anemia, and jaundice.

Maternal mortality rate: The maternal mortality rate is the number of maternal deaths per 100,000 women of reproductive age (15–49 years old).

MDG: Millennium Development Goals: Goals adopted in the Millennium Declaration at the General Assembly of the United Nations in September 2000. They focus on seven areas: Income Poverty, Food Security and Nutrition, Health and Mortality, Reproductive Health, Education, Gender Equality and Women's Empowerment, and the Environment.

MMR: A vaccine against measles, mumps, and rubella.

MMV: Medicines for Malaria Venture: A public-private partnership of global public health organizations, the pharmaceutical industry, government ministries, research institutions, and foundations that aims to develop new, effective, and affordable anti-malarial drugs.

Mortality rate: The per capita death rate in a population. (See also IMR, Maternal mortality rate, and Perinatal mortality rate.)

MRC: Medical Research Council: UK-based research organization that "aims to improve health by promoting research into all areas of medical and related science. It supports medical research in three main ways: through its research establishments; grants to individual scientists; and support for post graduate students." See http://www.mrc.ac.uk/

Multilateral agency: An agency involving more than two nations or parties. Multilateral lending agencies include the World Bank, the International Monetary Fund, and the Inter-American Development Bank.

NCD: Noncommunicable diseases: Diseases that cannot be transmitted between people (asthma, for example).

NCMH: National Commission on Macroeconomics and Health: A temporary official group within a developing country responsible for organizing and leading the task of scaling up health interventions, recommended by the Commission on Macroeconomics and Health. The NCMH, or its equivalent, would be chaired jointly by the Ministers of Health and Finance and would incorporate key representatives of civil society. The group would assess national health priorities, establish a multi-year strategy to extend coverage of essential health services, take account of synergies with other key health producing sectors, and ensure consistency with a sound macroeconomic policy framework. The plan would be predicated upon greatly expanded international grant assistance. The National Commission would work together with the WHO and World Bank to prepare an epidemiological baseline, quantified operational targets, and a medium-term financing plan.

NGO: Nongovernmental Organization: Private, nonprofit organizations that pursue activities to relieve suffering, promote the interests of the poor, protect the environment, provide basic social services, or undertake community development. NGOs often differ from other organizations in the sense that they tend to operate independently from government, are value-based, and are guided by the principles of altruism and voluntarism.

NIH: National Institutes of Health: One of eight agencies of the Public Health Services of the US Department of Health and Human Services. Conducts and supports research, trains researchers, and communicates medical information. See http://www.nih.gov

OCP: Onchocerciasis Control Programme: A WHO program to bring onchocerciasis (river blindness) under control in western Africa. See http://www.who.int/ocp/

ODA: Official Development Assistance: Development assistance of which at least 25 percent must be a grant or grant equivalent. The promotion of economic development or welfare must be the main objective. It must go to a developing country as defined by the DAC.

OECD: Organisation for Economic Co-operation and Development: An international organization, mainly of high-income countries, helping governments tackle the economic, social, and governance challenges of a globalized economy.

OI: Opportunistic Infection: Certain illnesses that people with AIDS can get and that can be life-threatening. People with healthy immune systems do not usually get these illnesses, even though most people have the organisms that cause these illnesses in their bodies already. Only when the immune system is damaged can the organism take advantage of the "opportunity" of this weakened state and cause damage.

OLIC: Other low-income countries: Countries other than LDCs with a per capita GNP of less than $765 in 1995, as listed in the DAC List of Aid Recipients used for the years 1997–1999.

Onchocerciasis: Onchocerciasis is also known as *river blindness* and is one form of filariasis (see Filariasis).

OPV: Oral polio vaccine.

Oral rehydration therapy: The treatment of diarrhea in which the patient drinks a special solution of salts and glucose to replace those lost as a result of the passage of loose, watery motion.

Orphan drug law: Orphan drugs are those developed under the US Orphan Drug Act (1983) to treat a disease that affects fewer than 200,000 people in the United States. The orphan drug law offers tax breaks and a 7-year monopoly on drug sales to induce companies to undertake the development and manufacturing of such drugs, which otherwise might not be profitable because of the small potential market.

Perinatal mortality rate: The number of intrauterine deaths after 28 weeks of gestation plus deaths in the first week of life divided by the total births. The rate is usually related to 1 year.

PIN: Population in need: The individuals that a disease prevention program or care intervention program is designed to reach.

Poverty trap: Persisting poverty.

PPP: Public-private partnership.

PPP $US: Purchasing Power Parity (adjusted dollars): A method of measuring the relative purchasing power of different countries' currencies over the same types of goods and services. Because goods and services may cost more in one country than in another, PPP allows us to make more accurate comparisons of standards of living across countries. PPP estimates use price comparisons of comparable items but since not all items can be matched exactly across countries and time, the estimates are not always "robust."

PRSP: Poverty Reduction Strategy Paper: Poverty Reduction Strategy Papers provide the basis for assistance from the World Bank and the International Monetary Fund as well as debt relief under the HIPC initiative. PRSPs should be country-driven, comprehensive in scope, partnership-oriented, and participatory. A country needs to write a PRSP only every 3 years. However, changes can be made to the content of a PRSP using an Annual Progress Report.

Public good: A public good has the properties of nonexcludability and nonrivalry. *Nonexcludability* implies that, when supplied, the direct and/or external benefits may not readily be denied to individuals or groups by requiring the payment of a fee or price. For example, the entire world community now benefits from elimination of small pox, and populations or countries could not be excluded from benefiting by instituting a fee. *Nonrivalry* implies that the consumption of the benefits of a good or service by an indivicual, group, or country will not diminish the benefit of others form the same good or service.

R&D: Research and development.

RIS: Residual insect spray: The main method of attacking adult mosquitoes in houses by spraying the inside surfaces of the walls and roof or ceiling with a residual insecticide. The intention is that mosquitoes will rest on the insecticide deposit and remain long enough to pick up a lethal dose.

Schistosomiasis: Schistosomiasis, also known as *bilharziasis* or *snail fever*, is a primarily tropical parasitic disease caused by the larvae of one or more of five types of flatworms or blood flukes known as schistosomes. There are five species of schistosomes that are prevalent in different areas of the world and produce somewhat different symptoms. Intestinal schistosomiasis, caused by *Schistosoma japonicum, S. mekongi, S. mansoni,* and *S. intercalatum,* can lead to serious complications of the liver and spleen. Urinary schistosomiasis is caused by *S. haematobium.* The World Health Organization (WHO) estimates that 200 million people are infected and 120 million display symptoms. Another 600 million people are at-risk of infection.

SWAp: Sector-wide approach: A strategy for development assistance in which a collective group of donor countries and a recipient country jointly plan, and commit to, a package of investments for a given sector (such as the health sector). In some cases a basket fund (a fund to support the entire package) is established into which participating donors contribute, and from which recipient countries make expenditures. The approach facilitates the integration of donor projects into the development plans of the recipient countries, enhances donor assistance coordination, promotes capacity building, and may increase the level of funding to hitherto neglected areas within a given sector.

STIs: Sexually transmitted infections: Infections that are passed from one person to another during sexual contact. This may include, but is not limited to, having intercourse. In some cases, any intimate skin-to-skin contact is sufficient for transmission of the infection to occur. Examples of STIs include HIV, chlamydia, gonorrhea, trichomoniasis, human papilloma virus (HPV), and herpes virus (HSV).

TB: Tuberculosis: A chronic or acute bacterial infection that primarily attacks the lungs, but that may also affect the kidneys, bones, lymph nodes, and brain. The disease is caused by *Mycobacterium tuberculosis,* a rod-shaped bacterium. Half of all untreated TB cases are fatal. Tuberculosis causes 2 million deaths a year. WHO predicts that between 2000 and 2020, nearly 1 billion people will become infected with the TB bacteria and 35 million people will die from the disease.

TDR: The Special Programme for Research and Training in Tropical Diseases (TDR): An independent global program of scientific collaboration. Established in 1975 and co-sponsored by the United Nations Development Programme (UNDP), the World Bank, and the World Health Organisation (WHO), it aims to help coordinate, support, and influence global efforts to combat a portfolio of ten major diseases of the poor and disadvantaged.

TRIPS: Trade-Related Aspects of Intellectual Property Rights. As part of the final Round (Uruguay Round) of the General Agreement on Tariffs and Trade (GATT) in April 1994, 123 countries signed the Agreement on Trade-Related Aspects of Intellectual Property Rights (TRIPS). It is an attempt to narrow the gaps in the way "intellectual property rights" (the right of creators to prevent others from using their inventions, designs, or other creations) are protected around the world. The TRIPS Agreement also brings them under common international rules. The TRIPS Agreement obliges all signatories to provide 20-year patent protection for novel, non-obvious inventions in all areas of technology, including pharmaceuticals. Enforcing resolutions under this agreement is the responsibility of the World Trade Organization (WTO).

Trypanosomiasis: A disease caused by trypanosomes, which are protozoan parasites. Infection by trypanosomes causes neurological alterations, leading to symptoms of chronic lethargy (hence the disease also called *African sleeping sickness*). Without treatment, the disease is invariably fatal. It is transmitted to humans through the bite of the tsetse fly of the genus *Glossina*. Sleeping sickness is a daily threat to more than 60 million men, women, and children in 36 countries of sub-Saharan Africa, 22 of which are among the least-developed countries in the world. Sleeping sickness has a major impact on the development of entire regions by decreasing the labor force and hampering production and work capacity.

UMIC: Upper-Middle-Income Countries. Countries that have per capita GDP income of between $US $2,996 and $9,265.

UN: United Nations: An international organization established in 1945 to preserve peace, solve international problems, and promote human rights through international cooperation and collective security. See http://www.un.org

UNDP: United Nations Development Program: The UN's principal provider of development advice, advocacy, and grant support. See http://www.undp.org

UNICEF: United Nations Children's Fund: A UN agency charged with advocating for children's rights and helping to meet their needs. See http://www.unicef.org

UNIDO: UN Industrial Development Organization: A UN agency that focuses its efforts on relieving poverty by fostering productivity growth in developing countries and countries with economies in transition. See http://www.unido.org

USAID: United States Agency for International Development: Independent federal government agency that works to support long-term and equitable economic growth and advance US foreign policy objectives by supporting economic growth and agricultural development, global health, and conflict prevention and developmental relief. See http://www.usaid.gov

User fees: Payment of out-of-pocket charges at the time of use of health care.

VCT: Voluntary counseling and testing.

Vector control: The elimination or containment of an organism (such as an insect) that transmits a causative agent (such as a bacterium or virus) of disease pathogen from one organism to another.

Vertical approach: Categorical approach to a particular disease.

VPD: Vaccine preventable disease.

WB: The World Bank: A development finance institution owned by 183 countries. The World Bank Group is one of the world's largest sources of development assistance, providing $17.3 billion in loans in FY2001. See http://www.worldbank.org

WHO: The World Health Organization: A specialized agency of the United Nations, focusing on health issues among its 191 Member States. WHO provides technical cooperation for health among nations, carries out programs to control and eradicate disease and strives to improve the quality of human life.

WTO: The World Trade Organization: "The only international organization dealing with the global rules of trade between nations. Its main function is to ensure that trade flows as smoothly, predictably, and freely as possible." See http://www.wto.org